Chiropractic:
The Greatest Hoax of the Century?

L.A. Chotkowski, MD, FACP

Second Edition © 2002
ISBN 0-9657855-2-8
Edited by Stephen Barrett, MD

New England Books
1143 Chamberlain Highway
Kensington, CT 06037
Tel. (860) 828-5016
Email: DrChot@aol.com

Contents

Part IV: Additional Perspectives

Part V: Appendices

About the Author

Ludmil Adam Chotkowski, MD, FACP, is a board-certified specialist in internal medicine who retired in 1986 after practicing medicine for 41 years. Born in Berlin, Connecticut, he was valedictorian of his high school class, graduated from Trinity College and Yale University School of Medicine, and completed his residency training at Hartford Hospital in Hartford, Connecticut. He then practiced privately for 25 years in Berlin, during which, at various times, he also served as a school physician, medical examiner, health director, medical staff president at New Britain Memorial Hospital, and an instructor at the University of Connecticut Medical School.

In his later years, Dr. Chotkowski served as Chief of Medicine at the Rocky Hill Veterans Home and Hospital and Medical Director of Connecticut State Mental Hospital. He is the author of several scientific medical articles published in the *New England Journal of Medicine*, the *Journal of the American Medical Association*, and *Connecticut Medicine*. He wrote a syndicated weekly newspaper column called "What's New in Medicine" for more than 30 years and in 1991 authored a book with the same name that won a Mosby book award. He also wrote a section on advances in medicine for the *Encyclopedia Americana*. In 1980, he received an American Cancer Society award for "excellence in communicating about cancer."

He is a member of the American Medical Association and the Connecticut State Medical Society and is a Fellow of the American College of Physicians (an honor awarded for his contributions to the practice of medicine).

Author's Dedication

This book is dedicated to the memory of my dear wife, Emily, who finally succumbed to an operation intended to mend the ravages of rheumatic heart disease on her mitral valve. She had a full life, sustained by a previous heart operation and the tender care of her doctors. I also wish to pay tribute to the men and women who have made the scientific medical discoveries that enable people to lead healthier, happier, and longer lives.

About the Editor

Stephen Barrett, MD, a retired psychiatrist who resides in Allentown, Pennsylvania, is a nationally renowned author, editor, and consumer advocate. He has been collecting information about chiropractic for more than 30 years. He is board chairman of Quackwatch, Inc.; vice president of the National Council Against Health Fraud; and editor of *Consumer Health Digest*, a free weekly e-mail newsletter. His 49 books include *The Health Robbers: A Close Look at Quackery in America; Reader's Guide to "Alternative" Health Methods;* and six editions of the college textbook *Consumer Health: A Guide to Intelligent Decisions*. He operates Quackwatch (www.quackwatch.com), Chirobase (www.chirobase.org), and six other Web sites. He can be reached at sbinfo@quackwatch.com or (610) 437-1795.

Acknowledgment

The author gives special thanks to freelance editor Sarah E. Fike, of Belleville, Illinois, who did a superb job of copy editing.

Part I
Overview

1
Why I Consider
Chiropractic a Hoax

Chiropractic is based on a century-old notion that spinal problems ("subluxations") are the cause or underlying cause of ill health. According to this notion: (a) vertebral "subluxations" press on spinal nerves and interfere with the passage of energy down those nerves to various organs, causing the organs to become diseased, and (b) spinal manipulation ("adjustments") can remedy these problems. Since this "discovery"—made by a grocer and "magnetic healer" in 1895—an entire profession has evolved, with some practitioners clinging to the original notion, some denouncing it, and others adopting a loosely defined middle ground. I consider these ideas, in all of their many forms, to be a hoax.

"Modern" Chiropractic

Chiropractic's most recent and "authoritative" description was formalized in 1996 by a consensus of the presidents of the 16 colleges forming the Association of Chiropractic Colleges (ACC). The resultant position paper stated the following, which I have slightly condensed:

> *ACC Position on Chiropractic*
> Chiropractic is a health care discipline which emphasizes the inherent recuperative power of the body to heal itself without the use of drugs or surgery.
>
> The practice of chiropractic focuses on the relationship between structure (primarily the spine) and function (as coordinated by the nervous system) and how

3

that relationship affects the preservation and restoration of health. In addition, Doctors of Chiropractic recognize the value and responsibility of working in cooperation with other health care practitioners when in the best interest of the patient. . . .

The Chiropractic Paradigm

The purpose of chiropractic is to optimize health.

The body's innate recuperative power is affected by and integrated through the nervous system.

The practice of chiropractic includes:

- Establishing a diagnosis;
- Facilitating neurological and biomechanical integrity through appropriate chiropractic case management; and
- Promoting health.

The foundation of chiropractic includes philosophy, science, art, knowledge, and clinical experience. . . .

The Subluxation

Chiropractic is concerned with the preservation and restoration of health, and focuses particular attention on the subluxation.

A subluxation is a complex of functional and/or structural and/or pathological articular changes that compromise neural integrity and may influence organ system function and general health.

A subluxation is evaluated, diagnosed, and managed through the use of chiropractic procedures based on the best available rational and empirical evidence.

Although the preceding statements are deliberately vague, they convey two themes that should be considered the basis of chiropractic today: (1) vertebral "subluxations" influence organ function and general health, and (2) managing them can preserve and restore health. These ideas clash with the body of basic knowledge of health, disease, and health care that scientists have developed through centuries of study.

VERTEBRAL SUBLUXATION AND NERVE CHART

This chart falsely suggests that misaligned spinal bones are the cause or underlying cause of earaches, gallbladder problems, liver problems, hardening of the arteries, pneumonia, crossed eyes, and scores of other health problems. Its listing in a recent catalog from chiropractic's leading supply house indicates that many chiropractors still exaggerate what spinal manipulation can do. (The details are intentionally blurred to avoid violating the publisher's copyright.)

My interest in chiropractic began during my childhood, as described in Chapter 2. During more than 40 years of medical practice, I encountered many patients whom chiropractors had mistreated for epilepsy, asthma, diabetes, cancer, and many other conditions for which they had nothing legitimate to offer. I eventually persuaded my state representative to introduce bills to the Connecticut legislature to prohibit or curtail certain chiropractic practices, including treatment of children, but these bills did not pass.

The final straw was a TV infomercial showing a chiropractor manipulating a newborn's neck and stating, "As the twig is bent, so grows the tree." This chiropractor advised mothers to have their babies' neck "subluxations" adjusted immediately after birth and subsequently throughout childhood in order to stay healthy. The chiropractor also advised against vaccinations. In my view, these activities amounted to a form of child abuse that should be challenged for what it is. During my investigation, I visited two chiropractic colleges, interviewed several chiropractors in depth, and sent and received correspondence from many more.

This book, the first such work written by a medical doctor, exposes fairly and honestly chiropractic's failure to prove that "adjusting" the spine can cure disease or maintain "wellness" or health in any way. The effectiveness of modern medicine against disease is well documented in standard medical texts. In contrast, no scientific proof exists for the claims that are central to chiropractic practice.

2
The Hoax in Action:
Three Cases

Many years ago, a 16-year-old high school student developed nausea that was accompanied by unusual abdominal pains. Her mother took her to the office of Dr. "X," whom a friend had recommended as particularly knowledgeable about female medical problems.

Dr. "X" treated the girl with abdominal massage and vigorous spinal manipulations. The mother thought this was strange. She did not object, however, because she believed that the doctor had been so highly recommended and therefore should be trustworthy. That night, the abdominal pain became so severe that the girl was rushed to a hospital where she was operated on for a ruptured appendix. Her postoperative course took several weeks, with life and death hanging in the balance.

After the operation, the mother was horrified to learn that she had taken her daughter to the wrong person. The expert her friend had recommended was a prominent medical doctor with the same name as a local chiropractor.

Acute appendicitis is usually easy to treat when diagnosed early. When permitted to fester, however, the appendix can burst and cause a severe infection (peritonitis) within the abdominal cavity. This, in turn, can lead to the development of bands of scar tissue (adhesions) that can strangulate the intestines. Although the girl survived, she developed adhesions and suffered from abdominal problems for the rest of her life.

I know this case well, for the girl was my sister. Although I was only 10 at the time, it launched my interest in chiropractic, which has culminated in the writing of this book.

My sister's chiropractor apparently believed that spinal misalignments ("subluxations") are the primary cause of ill health and that spinal manipulations are the remedy. This premise—still widely taught in chiropractic schools—can delay people from getting necessary medical care.

My Second Case

All through my premedical education at Trinity College and medical school at Yale, nothing was ever mentioned that I can recall about chiropractic. Perhaps something was said about the archaic homeopathic theory that "like cures like," meaning that substances that can cause symptoms can cure diseases with those symptoms when given in tiny amounts. Christian Science may also have been mentioned, but most medical students considered it unrealistic because it held that illness is an illusion and that medical care should be avoided. Yes, it seemed fine to pray for the sick—and certainly we planned to hope and pray for the recovery of our sick patients—but this did not involve the avoidance of medical care.

My fellow students and I knew that more medical research was needed and that we were the generation to carry on that quest for new knowledge.

So it was that my second encounter with chiropractic was a shocking experience. During my internship at Hartford Hospital, a man in his early 20s was brought into the emergency room unconscious, and I was called to examine him. The history was very sparse: Friends had found him unresponsive in his room and had him taken to the hospital by ambulance.

There was no evidence of head injury and no odor of alcohol on his breath, but his breath did smell sweet. He was in a deep coma and looked emaciated. His lips and tongue were extremely dry. His neck was flexible, which made it unlikely that he had meningitis or was bleeding from a ruptured aneurysm within the skull. The results of the neurologic examination were negative, except for the coma.

Among the possible causes of coma, diabetic acidosis seemed the most likely. Drug overdose was not as common as it is today, whereas diabetic coma was more so because the types of insulin back then were not as effective as those available today.

The diagnosis was quickly confirmed with blood tests that showed abnormally high levels of blood sugar and acetone and a deranged balance of electrolytes. So we administered 100 units of insulin intravenously along with a dilute salt-water solution to help restore his body fluid level and then planned to give more as needed based on his next blood sugar test and clinical findings. This regimen had been widely reported as effective and was considered state-of-the-art treatment at that time.

About half an hour after our treatment had begun, the man's distraught mother arrived and wanted to know what was happening. The conversation went something like this:

"Oh my God! What are you doing to him? My poor boy is dying. He won't answer me. What's in those bottles. He is unconscious. You know he has diabetes."

"We know," I assured her, "and we are giving him insulin, salt, and fluids. He is very seriously ill but is moving slightly and responding to treatment. He should make it."

"But how much insulin are you giving him. You know his doctor reduced his insulin dosage from 90 to 10 units a day. My son just hated to take his needles, and his doctor promised he would soon be able to stop taking the insulin entirely."

"Well, I just gave him 100 units and planned to give him another 100 units more, depending on his next blood sugar level in half an hour or so."

"My goodness, that's too much," she pleaded. "His doctor was massaging his pancreas and working on his back and had him down to 10 units."

"Madam, believe me, he needs the insulin," I advised, "and if he does not get it, he will certainly die.

Look, he is skin and bones and dry as the desert. His blood is all acid and his sugar is out of sight. If you don't like his treatment, you can take him elsewhere by signing him out against our advice, but I strongly feel we can save him if you would just be patient and trust us."

My firm reply seemed to have a calming effect, and the mother agreed to have him stay. I then asked what doctor was massaging his pancreas, manipulating his spine, and dropping his insulin dosage. It was a local chiropractor.

As the mother and I talked, the young man began to move about more and show signs of recovering—which he finally did, completely.

This incident happened in 1943 and, like my sister's unlucky encounter, was a consequence of faulty chiropractic theory. You might expect that irrational treatment like massaging an abdominal organ for a serious disease would not occur in modern times. Yet the next case shows that it does.

The Death of Andy Warhol

In February 1987, celebrity pop artist Andy Warhol died after surgical removal of his gallbladder. According to reports from the Associated Press and New York City's Chief Medical Examiner Dr. Elliot Gross, he died of a cardiac arrhythmia, as stated on the death certificate. Warhol's medical and autopsy records were private and available only to members of the deceased's family and could not be obtained for this book. However, the report Dr. Gross released to the press stated:

Regarding Andy Warhol, Case #M87-1718.

The investigation into the death of Andy Warhol, who died at the New York Hospital on February 22, 1987, has been concluded. Mr. Warhol had been admitted to the hospital for surgery on February 20, to remove an inflamed gallbladder due to a stone blocking the duct leading from the gallbladder.

The investigation included the autopsy, toxicological tests, a review of medical records and personal and telephone interviews with 30 individuals. One subpoena had to be issued.

The cause of death is a cardiac arrhythmia of undetermined origin following surgical removal of the gallbladder and repair of an abdominal incisional hernia under general anesthesia. In the absence of significant anatomical or toxicological findings, the cause of death is, therefore, a disturbance of the heart rhythm.

The findings of the autopsy on February 23rd and subsequent microscopic examination of tissues disclosed changes reflecting recent abdominal surgery. The operative site was intact and there was no internal hemorrhage.

There was mild atherosclerosis of the coronary arteries. The lumens of the coronary artery displayed no occlusion, significant narrowing or thrombosis. There was no anatomic evidence of other types of heart disease.

There was no pulmonary embolus. There were also no changes indicative of an allergic reaction.

Toxicologic tests on autopsy specimens detected prescribed drugs in concentrations consistent with their administration during and subsequent to surgery. Our microscopic examination of the gallbladder specimen indicated acute inflammation and longstanding chronic disease associated with gallstones. Our investigation also indicates that physical manipulation may have contributed to the onset of Mr. Warhol's immediate pre-hospital illness [1].

On March 1, 1987, the Associated Press reported on the case with the headline, "Warhol Complained of Pain after Visit to Chiropractor." The report stated:

Pop artist Andy Warhol complained of sharp pain after a chiropractor massaged his ailing gallbladder and tests later showed his condition had worsened and required prompt surgery, his doctors say.

Warhol died of a heart attack that occurred on the day after his operation. His problem grew from routine to acute surprisingly quickly, the doctor told the Associated Press. The doctor did not directly link the chiropractic treatment to the death of the 58-year-old Warhol, who emerged from surgery in stable condition but died the next morning, but he sharply criticized the massage.

"I am deeply concerned about it," said Dr. Denton Cox, who was Warhol's physician for 27 years. "It is inappropriate in the extreme for a nonprofessional to do it, and a professional person would not have done it."

Dr. Karen Burke, Warhol's dermatologist and a friend, said Warhol described the massage to her as a "mashing" of his gallbladder. The chiropractor, Linda Li, declined comment on the matter when reached by telephone at her office. After learning the purpose of the call, she said, "I think I'll conclude the conversation at this time" and hung up.

Louis Sportelli, a chiropractor and a board member of the American Chiropractic Association, rejected any connection of the treatment to Warhol's worsened condition. He said organ massage is too gentle to have such an effect, but he also said that the practice is not widely accepted in the chiropractic community.

"To relate the chiropractic manipulation or massage of that gallbladder to the ultimate consequence of what happened is ridiculous," Sportelli said Saturday. He said that linking the massage to Warhol's death was "stretching to place blame where none exits," and suggested it could "stem from prejudice by medical doctors against chiropractors." [2]

Sportelli's response—blaming criticim of chiropractic on medical bias—is one of the typical ways chiropractors defend themselves. Yet mashing a diseased gallbladder is a ridiculous thing to do. The gallbladder, when diseased or filled with stones, can become swollen. In this state, it may be felt by the hand and be accessible to massage. However, massage is dangerous because it can cause or increase inflammation, which can lead to rupture. No competent medical doctor would do such a thing.

Sportelli did not say why the chiropractor massaged Warhol's gallbladder or whether she also manipulated his spine. Why didn't the press ask him to explain exactly what chiropractors can do for gallbladder disease and provide evidence that would justify any such claim?

Death caused by senseless treatment can result in criminal prosecution, but such cases are rare. The most famous one occurred about 40 years ago when a chiropractor was convicted of second-degree murder after he persuaded the parents of an 8-year-old girl with cancer to permit him to treat her with vitamins and spinal manipulation instead of standard medical treatment [3]. But Andy Warhol's chiropractor was not prosecuted.

During the 1970s, Palmer College published about 50 pamphlets promoting chiropractic for appendicitis, diabetes, gallbladder disease, and many other health problems. Although these pamphlets are no longer sold, other publishers still sell many pamphlets that proclaim that "subluxations" can cause ill health throughout the body and that spinal "adjustments" can fix them.

On August 1, 1987, *The New York Times* reported that no criminal charge would be brought because the exact relationship between the chiropractor's treatment and the cause of death could not be determined [4].

Why Danger Persists

These three cases illustrate how chiropractic's failure to limit its scope can have extremely serious consequences. The percentage of chiropractors who would attempt to treat appendicitis, diabetic acidosis, an inflamed gallbladder, and other conditions requiring urgent medical care is unknown. The percentage is probably not high and is certainly lower than it was decades ago. However, widespread beliefs that spinal "adjustments" may help problems throughout the body still encourage chiropractors to use it inappropriately.

References

1. Press release, Office of the Chief Medical Examiner, New York City.
2. Associated Press. Warhol complained of pain after visit to chiropractor. New York Times, March 1, 1987.
3. Smith RL. At Your Own Risk: The Case against Chiropractic. New York: Pocket Books, 1969.
4. New York Times, August 1, 1987.

3
NCAHF Fact Sheet
on Chiropractic (2001)

Chiropractic is a controversial health care system that originated in the United States in 1895. The National Council Against Health Fraud (NCAHF) finds it remarkable that the chiropractic profession has existed for a century without having made a single notable contribution to the world's body of knowledge in the health sciences. The reason for this failure can be found in its origins and in the continued presence of antiscience attitudes. This includes the fields of the care and prevention of back pain and the value of spinal manipulative therapy (SMT), the areas in which chiropractic has dominated the health care services marketplace. Recent pronouncements on the value of manipulative therapy for back pain have involved medical research, not work done by doctors of chiropractic (DCs). DC publicists have been quick to grab the credit for these findings for marketing purposes, but deserve little credit. Some research projects are now under way, but chiropractic still does not play a significant role in researching the causes and treatment of the human ailments from which it derives most of its income.

In the Beginning . . .

Chiros (hand) + *practos* (practice) literally means "done by hand." Chiropractic was invented in 1895 by Daniel D. Palmer, a layperson in Davenport, Iowa [1]. Because he sold goldfish commercially, Palmer is referred to by some historians as a "fish monger." It is more interesting to know that he practiced magnetic healing beginning in the mid-1880s in Burlington, Iowa. Palmer searched for the single cause of all disease. The standard story about chiropractic's "discovery" is that Palmer believed he had found the single cause of disease when he "cured" the deafness of janitor Harvey Lillard by manipulating his spine. (Palmer may have learned spinal manipulation from Andrew Still's osteopathic school in Kirksville, Missouri). Lillard is said to have lost his hearing while working in a cramped, stooped position during which he felt something snap in his back.

Palmer's version of this event has always been disputed by Lillard's daughter, Valdeenia Lillard Simons. She says that her father told her that he was telling jokes to a friend in the hall outside Palmer's office and, Palmer, who had been reading, joined them. When Lillard reached the punch line, Palmer, laughing heartily, slapped Lillard on the back with the hand holding the heavy book he had been reading. A few days later, Lillard told Palmer that his hearing seemed better. Palmer then decided to explore manipulation as an expansion of his magnetic healing practice. Simons said "the compact was that if they can make [something of] it, then they both would share. But, it didn't happen." [2]

Chiropractic's true origin appears to have been of a more mystical nature than the Lillard tale denotes. Palmer was an active spiritualist and apparently believed that the idea of "replacing displaced vertebrae for the relief of human ills" came in a spiritualist séance through communication with the spirit of Dr. Jim Atkinson, a physician who had died 50 years earlier in Davenport [3]. As a young man, Palmer regularly walked the six or seven miles to the estate of his spiritualist mentor, William Drury [4]. It was one of Drury's followers who told him of her vision of a door with a sign on it reading "Dr. Palmer." She said that he one day would lecture in a large hall telling an audience about a new "revolutionary" method of healing the sick [5]. Predisposed to magnetic healing by his belief in spiritualism, Palmer was drawn to the practice by seeing the financial success of illiterate "Dr." Paul Caster of Ottumwa. Palmer's grandson described his technique:

He would develop a sense of being positive within his own body; sickness being negative. He would draw his hands over the area of the pain and with a sweeping motion stand aside, shaking his hands and fingers vigorously, taking away the pain as if it were drops of water [6].

Palmer began speculating that the flow of animal magnetism may become blocked by obstructions along the spine [7]. Palmer taught that chiropractic was "an educational, scientific, religious system" that "associates its practice, belief and knowledge with that of religion" and "imparts instruction relating both to this world and the world to come." "Chiropractic," Palmer stated, "sheds enlightenment upon physical life and spiritual existence, the latter being only a continuation of the former." [8] Individual chiropractors sometimes deny that they believe in Palmer's biotheological "Innate Intelligence," but when pressed as to their basis for practice, they must face the physiological facts described in a scientific brief on chiropractic:

> If there is partial blockage of impulses in a nerve fibre
> . . . the impulse is transmitted more slowly in a zone of
> partial blockage, and resumes all its characteristics as
> soon as it reaches normal tissue. Thus, it is impossible
> for a partial blockage of nerve impulses in a particular
> zone to affect the flow, since the impulses would re-
> sume their normal flow [9].

Unsupported by science, chiropractors must either fall back on Palmer's pantheistic views or admit that the "subluxation" theory is erroneous. Without this theory, chiropractors are reduced to spinal manipulators whose primary treatment modality is shared by osteopaths, physiatrists, sports trainers, physical therapists, and others. Without subluxation theory, chiropractic's claim that it is a unique and comprehensive "alternative" to standard medicine is lost. D.D. Palmer had only modest success in promoting chiropractic. It was his son, B.J. Palmer, an eccentric promoter and Iowa radio industry pioneer, who developed chiropractic into a successful business enterprise.

Vitalistic Theory

According to fundamentalist chiropractic theory, spinal "subluxations" mechanically interfere with nerve flow (the "Innate Life Force"), weakening organs served by the nerves and making them more susceptible to disease. Thus:

> "Subluxations" are the primary "cause" of disease, and restoration of nerve flow is essential to healing.
>
> The "Innate" is said to represent 'Universal Intelligence' (God); the function of 'Innate Intelligence' (Soul, Spirit or Spark of Life) within each, which D.D. Palmer considered a minute segment of 'Universal.'
>
> The fundamental causes of interference to the planned expression of that Innate Intelligence are Mental, Chemical and/ or Mechanical Stresses that create the structural distortions that interfere with nerve supply [10].

Appeal

Chiropractic combines metaphysical and mechanistic explanations of health and disease in a simplistic fashion. DCs have repeatedly outperformed other providers in assessments of patient satisfaction [11-13]. DCs mostly treat back pain and are more sympathetic and supportive of patients' complaints. To DCs, back problems are significant to overall health, whereas physicians consider such problems minor and self-limiting.

Census

The American Chiropractic Association (ACA) estimates that there are between 55,000 and 70,000 chiropractors in the United States [14]. *Dynamic Chiropractic*, a newspaper sent to every chiropractor it can locate, circulates to about 60,000 chiropractors in the United States, including 10,000 in California [15]— the most in any state.

Legal Status

All 50 states and the District of Columbia attempt to regulate chiropractic via licensure. DCs are also licensed in several other countries. One of the most difficult aspects of regulating chiropractors is the ambiguity of their legally defined scope of practice. Most health care providers are limited to some precisely delineated structure or function of the body. For instance, dentists are limited to treating the oral cavity, podiatrists are limited to treating the feet, and optometrists are limited to correcting vision problems. Chiropractors are limited to analyzing and manipulating the back, but this is no limit at all if you accept the chiropractic paradigm, which holds that nerve "energy" is a metaphysical entity that travels from out of the cosmos, into the mind, down through the spine, and into every organ of the body and that chiropractors can detect interferences with that cosmic energy flow and restore full power through manipulation or other methods. Chiropractors allege that virtually all health problems may be affected by their "adjustments." They also assert that they can treat any condition that may benefit from improving the flow of an alleged cosmic energy that emanates either from the throne of God or the nucleus of the Big Bang—depending on one's fundamental beliefs. Limiting the scope of practice of ideological, nonmedical providers is the key to a great deal of consumer protection, but the practical problems of doing so can be confusing [16].

Factionalism

To understand the confused world of chiropractic, one must differentiate between chiropractic theory (aka, "philosophy") and chiropractic practitioner factions. Chiropractic is a conglomeration of factions in conflict. Most obvious is the dichotomy of "straights" versus "mixers," who are represented by two separate national organizations, the International Chiropractors Association and the ACA, respectively. At least a dozen different notions about how the spine should be corrected divide DCs. A government report has described the chaos within chiropractic:

> Heated controversy regarding chiropractic theory and practice continues to exist. On-site and telephone discussions with chiropractors and their schools and associations, coupled with a review of background materials . . . result in a picture of a profession in transition and containing a number of contradictions. There continues to be some disagreement with the profession regarding which conditions are appropriate for chiropractic care and regarding appropriate parameters for treatment [17].

Scientific Status

Chiropractic theory has failed tests of both validity and reliability. The "subluxation," which is the foundation of its theory, has never been demonstrated to exist. Moreover, anatomist Edmund Crelin, PhD, twisted cadaver spines and found that nerves were not impinged as chiropractors postulate [18].

The ACA is equivocal on the idea of the existence and importance of spinal misalignments [19]. DCs have repeatedly failed field tests of reliability. Chiropractic public relations have exaggerated the significance of a British study that compared the satisfaction of patients with low back pain (screened for contraindications to manipulation) who received private practice DC care with others who were treated by physiotherapists in the government's Royal Hospital Service [13].

Chiropractors often misrepresent a review of manipulative therapy by the Rand Corporation [20,21] as proof of chiropractic's value. They generally do not reveal that:

- The Rand study was not conducted because of some new indication of the apparent scientific merit of manipulative therapy, but because the chiropractic profession paid to have the study done.

- Four of the nine evaluators of the studies were chiropractors who were favorably biased toward manipulation.
- Only four of the 22 controlled trials they evaluated involved chiropractic care. The others involved safer techniques used by physical therapists, DOs, etc.
- The Rand panel concluded that "the efficacy of spinal manipulation is neither proven nor disproven at this time."

A 1993 report by a Canadian economist, Pran Manga, who is a satisfied chiropractic patient, declared that chiropractic was safer, more effective, and more cost-effective than medical management of low back pain [22], but these conclusions were refuted by Rand's Dr. Paul Shekelle who noted that Manga had looked at "the exact same studies as the rest of us, and no one else has been able to come to those conclusions." [23] The Manga report was also severely criticized by Dr. Hamilton Hall, director of the Canadian Back Institute [24].

The Rand Corporation also reviewed the appropriateness of manipulation and mobilization of the cervical spine, employing the same technique it had used to evaluate SMT for back pain. Only 11.1% of 736 indications for cervical manipulation were judged appropriate by a panel of nine judges (four DCs, four MDs, and one MD-DC). The most important finding was the paucity of evidence for the benefit of these procedures [25]. The risks of cervical spine manipulation are well documented. (For details on workers compensation and other studies involving chiropractic treatment of back pain, see the NCAHF consumer information statement on chiropractic back care.)

Antitrust Legal Victory

DCs won a highly publicized antitrust lawsuit in 1987. Chiropractic public relations messages have largely misrepresented its significance. The facts of the case help put it in proper perspective. From 1966 to 1980, the American Medical Association's (AMA) code of ethics prohibited its members from collaborating with DCs. The change in 1980 apparently resulted from legal advice and not because the AMA felt that DCs had become acceptable. In 1976, several DCs filed an antitrust lawsuit (*Wilk v AMA, et al*) charging restraint of trade under the Sherman Antitrust Act, a law designed to ensure marketplace competition.

The AMA was acquitted in 1981, but the case was overturned on appeal. In the new trial, the plaintiffs asked only for an injunction to prohibit the AMA from ever again imposing an ethical restriction on its members to refer patients to DCs. The Sherman Act was meant to apply business, not to scientific affairs. An important legal question involved whether the AMA's ethical prohibition had been exempt from the Sherman Act. The AMA argued that the scientific aspects of patient care had been their reason for prohibiting members from collaboration. In 1987, Judge Susan Getzendanner decided that the AMA's concerns had been justified and were the dominating factor in its behavior (rather than economics). Nevertheless, she found the AMA guilty because it had failed to prove that its ethical boycott was reasonable and the least restrictive of competition.

Once the ethical boycott was determined to have been illegal, chiropractic propagandists labeled it a "conspiracy" and proclaimed that the AMA was found guilty of conspiring to eliminate chiropractic. Their message implies that the "conspiracy" was secret and medically unjustified and that the court's finding proved that chiropractic is a valid health care system. None of these is true. Judge Getzendanner stated that her ruling had no bearing on the validity of chiropractic and that the ethical boycott was done openly.

It must be noted that MDs are not required to refer patients to DCs and that referring physicians assume some risk for harm that comes to patients at the hands of practitioners to whom they were referred, particularly if there was reason to fear that the practitioner uses unscientific practices. Since some DCs reject cultism and pseudoscience, DCs must be evaluated on an individual basis. (See also: "Statement from AMA's General Counsel." *JAMA* 259:83, 1988)

Major Risks

Forceful neck manipulations can cause stroke and paralysis. A survey by the Stanford (University) Stroke Center found that within a 2-year period, 56 strokes had occurred among patients within 24 hours after receiving neck manipulation by a DC. One patient died, and 86% were left with permanent impairment. Most cases involved intervertebral artery damage. The age range of patients affected was 21 to 60 years, with most occurring in young individuals [26]. The Manitoba College of Physicians and Surgeons advised doctors to warn patients about the risks of neck manipulation after it was found that six cases of brainstem injury resulting in permanent paralysis had occurred within the province in the previous 3 years. Manitoba has a population of about 1 million, and since not all go to DCs, such an incidence of injury greatly exceeds the estimated 1-in-10 million risk associated with such procedures [27]. A bibliography of 166 documented and 17 anecdotal reports of vertebrobasilar injury after SMT was published in 1996 [28].

Full-spine x-ray exposure of the type used by many DCs may cause cancer. Dosimetric calculations used to test the theory that full-spine x-rays help detect bony neoplasms, both a contraindication to manipulation of the spine and an early detection of cancer, led to the conclusion that a full-spine x-ray of a 25-year-old male is twice as likely to cause the patient's death from cancer than it is to detect a bony tumor [29]. A five-view lumbosacral series of x-rays exposes the gonads to 3,000 times more radiation than front-to-back and lateral chest x-rays. The National Academy of Sciences Research Council estimates that spinal radiography causes an estimated 100 to 200 deaths per year from various cancers [30].

Indirect harm attributable to chiropractors includes improper treatment as a result of failure to diagnose a condition [31,32] and the practice of many chiropractors to discourage parents from immunizing their children based on chiropractic philosophy [33–35].

In 1994, the chiefs of the departments of pediatrics and pediatric hospitals in Canada issued the following statement:

> We wish to express our great concern over unscientific claims being made by Canadian chiropractors regarding the proper care of infants and children. These claims come from official statements from both the Canadian and Ontario Chiropractic Associations. Chiropractic treatment for such conditions as ear infections, infantile colic, newborn jaundice, spinal scoliosis and tonsillitis, amongst others, are being recommended in at least one major textbook being used at the Canadian Memorial Chiropractic College in Toronto. We call upon the governments of Ontario and Quebec, which have the only two chiropractic schools in Canada, to evaluate the courses being taught and the claims being made by the graduates of these schools regarding the treatment of infants and children. Contrary to the information being provided to parents and to the general public:
>
> 1. Chiropractic spinal manipulation is NOT required as a preventive therapy to maintain a child's health.
>
> 2. Chiropractic spinal manipulation is NOT an alternative for pediatric immunization. Books sold at the Canadian Memorial Chiropractic College in Toronto are anti-immunization in nature.
>
> 3. Chiropractic does NOT alter the course of, nor does it prevent in any way, childhood illness such as ear infections, asthma attacks, bed-wetting, or infantile colic.
>
> 4. Chiropractic use of x-rays of infants and children to diagnose so called vertebral subluxations is unscientific and of no value whatsoever. These x-rays can contribute, without any benefit to the child, to the future risk in the child of cancers and genetic damage. Parents should never allow their children's spines to be x-rayed by a chiropractor.

5. There is no scientific evidence whatsoever that the so-called chiropractic spinal adjustment results in any correction to a child's spine. These adjustments are ineffective and useless.

6. School boards should not authorize, and parents should not allow their children to attend, elementary school screening programs organized by chiropractors to detect scoliosis or any other postural deformities in children. Postural deformities of children such as scoliosis, kyphosis, or unequal leg lengths are not effectively treated by manipulation. In the great majority of instances, what a chiropractor may diagnose as scoliosis in a child is in fact a minor variation in a perfectly normal spine.

7. Parents should regard with extreme skepticism claims made by some other parents that their infants or children have been cured by chiropractic adjustments for such conditions as infant colic, recurrent ear infections, learning disorders, asthma, chronic abdominal cramps, or bed-wetting. However well meaning, such personal testimony is unreliable and is not a substitute for scientific fact.

Parents should read the June 1994 issue of *Consumer Reports* magazine in which the clear recommendation is made not to allow any chiropractor to solicit children for chiropractic treatment.

8. We understand the concern of parents in regard to ear infections that they may feel their child has taken many antibiotics or may require a surgical procedure. These concerns should not lead the parents to believe that chiropractic adjustments, which have the emotional appeal of being medication free or "natural" are an alternative to what may very well be in the best overall interests of the child.

9. We welcome the scientific guidelines of the Orthopractic Manipulation Society International, under which manual therapy can be given in a responsible manner to adults who may require such care. We welcome warnings made in these guidelines about the unscientific use of x-rays and unscientific claims about treating pediatric conditions. We would encourage parents to seek their own personal care from their physical therapists, physicians, and chiropractors who adhere to the scientific guidelines of the Orthopractic Manipulation Society International.

10. The musculo-skeletal problems of infants and children can be managed in a safe, scientific, and responsible manner by the family physician, the orthopedic specialist, the physical therapist, and with medical consultation, those chiropractors who adhere to the orthopractic guidelines.

11. We believe it to be irresponsible, and a total waste of our limited financial resources for the governments of Ontario, Manitoba, Saskatchewan, Alberta and British Columbia to be providing millions of dollars of public funds for chiropractors to treat infants and children. This public fiscal support gives parents the false impression that society endorses the treatments. We call upon these governments to immediately suspend all chiropractic payments in the pediatric age group, i.e., up to 18 years [36].

Chiropractic Treatment of Childrens' Asthma. After a 3-week baseline evaluation, 91 children who had continuing symptoms of asthma despite usual medical therapy were randomly assigned to receive either active or simulated chiropractic manipulation (tantamount to placebo treatment) for 4 months. None had previously received chiropractic care. Each subject was treated by 1 of 11 participating DCs selected by parents according to location. The primary outcome measure was the change from baseline in the peak expiratory flow that was measured in the morning before the use of a bronchodilator at 2 and 4 months. Except for the treating DC and one investigator (who was not involved in assessing outcomes), all participants remained fully blinded to the treatment assignment throughout the study. The researchers found no significant differences in improvements between the two groups [37].

Chiropractic Reformers

In 1987, chiropractors who reject the metaphysical biotheology and antimedical attitudes of chiropractic but see value in manipulative therapy for limited conditions organized the National Association for Chiropractic Medicine (NACM) [38]. NACM practitioners focus on the conservative treatment of musculoskeletal conditions. Manual therapy is their main treatment, but the use of drugs such as pain relievers and muscle relaxants is considered desirable if they are legally available. NACM's open rejection of the subluxation theory and chiropractic philosophy and its acceptance of the scientific method set it apart from other factions within the chiropractic guild. This also has made it the target of scorn by chiropractic's true believers.

In 1994, NACM announced that it was giving up its struggle to reform mainstream chiropractic and was joining with an international group of manipulative therapists called orthopractors. NACM would become a U.S. chapter of the Orthopractic Manipulation Society (OMS) [23,39]. Orthopractic therapy involves restoring a greater range of motion to the joints of the body through gentle and gradual mobilization or more forceful manipulation. Among other things, orthopractors (a) provide patient education that is aimed at reducing pain and disability and having the patients become independent of care; (b) specifically reject the chiropractic subluxation theory; (c) do not use x-rays in diagnosis; (d) reject the use of manipulation to treat postural deformities in children (e.g., kyphosis, scoliosis, unequal leg lengths) or a variety of children's ailments (e.g., colic, eczema, learning disorders, infections, asthma, and more); (e) reject spinal manipulations for general health care; (f) support immunization; (g) reject the use of testimonials to promote their services; (h) reject homeopathy; and (i) advise against sales promotions by chiropractors such as family plans, lifelong spinal adjustments, free x-ray examinations, and elementary school screening programs for scoliosis [40].

In addition to organizing like-minded practitioners, establishing a new profession requires the passage of new practices acts by state legislatures, the development of education and training programs, and the marketing of the profession in a competitive setting. Political resistance to reform by traditional DCs and organized chiropractic is strong. The idea of an orthopractic profession was such a serious threat to chiropractic in the United States that state licensing boards threatened to discipline chiropractors who identify themselves as orthopractors. The organizational effort was squelched because orthopractors lacked the resources to simultaneously organize a new profession and defend against aggressive legal actions in state after state. Despite its inability to establish an evidence-based guild of manipulative therapy practitioners in the United States, orthopractic made its mark by describing what a legitimate profession would look like.

The Future of Chiropractic

At least 70% of adults will experience low back pain (LBP) at some time in their lives. Back symptoms usually begin in the third or fourth decade of life, peak on incidence in the 40s and early 50s, and decline rapidly thereafter. There has been no sex differences in incidence noted. Although acute LBP is a self-limiting illness, it can persist for a considerable time [41]. The main advantage of SMT is that it can provide more rapid relief in about one third of patients. There is more information on the value of manipulation by non-DCs than there is for DCs. However, NCAHF believes that our society has sufficient need for preventing (through ergonomics) and treating back pain (by manipulative therapy and medication) to sustain limited-scope health care providers under the entitlement of "chiropractors." This will require greater attention to scientific research on the appropriate applications of SMT, expanding chiropractic training to include pharmacology, and rewriting state chiropractic practice acts to limit their scope of practice. Western States Chiropractic College (Portland, Oregon) is working in this direction and has changed the name of its diploma to "Doctor of Chiropractic Medicine." Sectarian DCs are objecting vociferously to this advancement toward science. Precisely what will become of chiropractic in the future is uncertain. NCAHF believes that as some factions become more scientific, antiscientific chiropractic groups will continue to exist within chiropractic until it becomes economically impossible for them to survive.

Consumer Beware

B.J. Palmer considered chiropractic to be a business, not a profession. He advised DCs to advertise and to sell their patients on the philosophy of chiropractic. Chiropractic education is proprietary (i.e., a business of its own). Unlike physicians, DCs do not go into residency programs after graduation. They are dumped on the marketplace to survive by whatever means necessary. Having been taught to be entrepreneurs, many sell whatever they can to make money. DCs regularly invade fields of health care in which they have no real skill (e.g., dietetics, physical therapy, sports medicine, pediatrics, and even veterinary medicine). Despite the obvious conflict of interest involved, many DCs sell dietary supplements, homeopathic remedies, herbal remedies, and other items directly to their patients. DCs take formal courses in practice-building that teach methods of deception. Consumers are often no match for the schemes and scams DCs invent.

References

1. Beck BL. Magnetic healing, spiritualism ... chiropractic: Palmer's union of methodologies. Chiropractic History 11(2):11–16, 1991.
2. Westbrooks B. The troubled legacy of Harvey Lillard: the black experience in chiropractic. Chiropractic History 2(1)46–53, 1982.
3. Palmer DD. Textbook of the Science, Art and Philosophy of Chiropractic. Portland Printing House, 1910, pp. 11–12.
4. Gielow V. Old Dad Chiro: Biography of D.D. Palmer. Davenport, IA: Bauder Brothers, 1981, p. 26.
5. Maynard J. Healing Hands. Mobile, AL: Jonorm Publishing, 1981, p. 10.
6. Palmer, David Daniel. The Palmers: A Pictorial Life Story. Davenport, IA: Bauder Brothers (undated), p. 76.
7. Fuller R. Alternative Medicine and American Religious Life. New York: Oxford University Press, 1989, p. 69.
8. Palmer DD. The Chiropractor. Los Angeles: Beacon Light, 1914, p. 4.
9. College of Physicians and Surgeons of the Province of Quebec. A scientific brief against chiropractic. The New Physician, Sept 1966.
10. Homewood AE. The Neurodynamics of the Vertebral Subluxation. St. Petersburg, FL: Valkyrie Press, 1973.
11. Kane RL and others. Manipulating the patient; comparison of the effectiveness of physician and chiropractic care. Lancet 1:1333–1336, 1974.
12. Cherkin D, MacCornack F. Patient evaluations of low back pain care family physicians and chiropractors. Western Journal of Medicine 150:351–355, 1989.
13. Meade TW and others. Low back pain of mechanical origin: Randomized comparison of chiropractic and hospital outpatient treatment. British Medical Journal 300:1431–1437, 1990.
14. Frequently asked questions. American Chiropractic Association Web site, accessed October 31, 2001.
15. Circulation breakdown. Dynamic Chiropractic, April 9, 2001.
16. Cohen MH. Scope of practice limitations on unconventional providers: The case of chiropractic. Alternative and Complementary Therapies, March–April 1996, pp. 110–114.
17. Inspection of Chiropractic Services Under Medicare. Chicago: Department of Health and Human Services, Office of Analysis, Aug 1986.
18. Crelin EM. A scientific test of the chiropractic theory. American Scientist 61:574–580, 1973.
19. Chiropractic: State of the Art 1994-1995. Arlington, VA: American Chiropractic Association, 1994.
20. The Appropriateness of Spinal Manipulation for Low-Back Pain, Project Overview and Literature Review. Santa Monica, CA: Rand Corp, 1991.
21. Shekelle PG. RAND misquoted. ACA Journal of Chiropractic 30(7):59–63, 1993.
22. Manga P and others. The Effectiveness and Cost-Effectiveness of Chiropractic Management of Low-Back Pain. Richmond Hill, Ontario, Canada: Kenelworth Publishing, 1993.

23. Chiropractors. Consumer Reports 59:383–390, 1994.
24. Lowry F. Orthopedists have bone to pick with economist over report on chiropractic. Canadian Medical Association Journal 150:1878–1881, 1994.
25. Coulter ID and others. The Appropriateness of Manipulation and Mobilization of the Cervical Spine. Santa Monica, CA: Rand Corporation, 1996.
26. Lee KP and others. Neurological complications following chiropractic manipulation: A survey of California neurologists. Neurology 45:1213–1215, 1995.
27. Brosnahan M. After six paralyzed in Manitoba, college warns neck manipulation dangerous. The Medical Post, Jan 28, 1986, p. 23.
28. Terett AGJ. Vertebrobasilar Stroke Following Manipulation. West Des Moines, IA: National Chiropractic Mutual Insurance Company, 1996.
29. Fickel TE. An analysis of the carcinogenicity of full spine radiography. ACA Journal of Chiropractic 23(5):61–66, 1986.
30. Hockberger RS. Meeting the challenge of low back pain. Emergency Medicine, Aug 15, 1990, p. 99.
31. Nickerson HJ and others. Chiropractic manipulation and children. Journal of Pediatrics 121:172, 1992.
32. Modde PJ. Malpractice is an inevitable result of chiropractic philosophy and training. Legal Aspects of Medical Practice, Feb 1979, pp. 20–24.
33. Nelson CA. Why chiropractors should embrace immunization. ACA Journal of Chiropractic, May 1993, pp. 79–85.
34. WCA adds legal action to immunization arsenal. The Chiropractic Journal 6(5):1, 1992.
35. Gunter GT. Immunization: A review for chiropractors. Today's Chiropractic, Sept–Oct 1986, pp. 15–18.
36. Haslam RHA and others. Statement of the chiefs of the departments of pediatrics of pediatric hospitals in Canada. Aug 19, 1994.
37. Balon J and others: A comparison of active and simulated chiropractic manipulation as adjunctive treatment for childhood asthma. New England Journal of Medicine 339:1013–1020, 1998.
38. Slaughter R. Chiropractors want new profession. Medical World News, Aug 10, 1987, p. 58.
39. NACM seeks to create new profession: Orthopractors. Dynamic Chiropractic, May 20, 1994.
40. Orthopractic Manipulation Society of North America (pamphlet). Beaconsfield, Quebec, Canada, 1994.
41. Croft PR and others. Outcome of low back pain in general practice: A prospective study. British Medical Journal 316:1356–1359, 1998.

Part II

What Others Have Said

H.L. Mencken Debunks Chiropractic

At Your Own Risk: The Case against Chiropractic

The Views of *Consumer Reports*

Smart Money Hits a Raw Nerve

The Lemmon/Matthau Takeoff

4

H.L. Mencken
Dubunks Chiropractic (1924)

Henry Louis Mencken (1880-1956) was a controversial American journalist, essayist, and literary critic. During the 1920s, he became famous for his vitriolic attacks on what he considered to be the hypocrisy, stupidity, and bigotry of much of American life. His critics considered him highly skilled at satire but intolerant and often crude. The following essay was published in the *Baltimore Evening Sun* in December 1924. Although the medical knowledge of his day was still quite primitive, Mencken knew enough to realize that chiropractic theory was a hoax. A more modern version of chiropractic ridicule is described in Chapter 8.

Chiropractic

This preposterous quackery is now all the rage in the back reaches of the Republic and even begins to conquer the less civilized of the big cities. As the old-time family doctor dies out in the country towns, with no trained successor willing to take over his dismal business, he is followed by some hearty blacksmith or ice-wagon driver, turned into a chiropractor in six months, often by correspondence.

In Los Angeles the damned, there are more chiropractors than actual physicians and they are far more generally esteemed. Proceeding from the Ambassador Hotel to the heart of the town, along Wilshire Boulevard, one passes scores of their gaudy signs; there are even many chiropractic "hospitals." The morons who pour in from the prairies and deserts, most of them ailing, patronize these "hospitals" copiously, and give to the chiropractic pathology the same high respect that they accord to the theology of Aimee McPherson and the art of Cecil De Mille. That pathology is grounded upon the doctrine that all human ills are caused by the pressure of misplaced vertebrae upon the nerves which come out of the spinal cord—in other words, that every disease is the result of a pinch. This plainly enough is buncombe. The chiropractic therapeutics rest upon the doctrine that the way to get rid of such pinches is to climb upon a table and submit to an heroic pummeling by a retired piano mover. This, obviously, is buncombe doubly damned.

Both doctrines were launched upon the world by an old quack named Andrew T. Still, the father of osteopathy. For years his followers merchanted them, and made a lot of money at the trade. But as they grew opulent, they grew ambitious, i.e., they began to study anatomy and physiology. The result was a gradual abandonment of Papa Still's ideas. The high-toned osteopathy of today is a sort of eclectic. He tries anything that promises to work, from tonsillectomy to the vibrations of the late Dr. Abrams. With four years' training behind him, he probably knows more anatomy than the average graduate of the John Hopkins Medical School or, at all event, more osteology. Thus enlightened, he seldom has much to say about pinched nerves in the back. But as he abandoned the Still revelation, it was seized by the chiropractors, led by another quack, one Palmer. This Palmer grabbed the pinched nerve nonsense and began teaching it to ambitious farmhands and out-at-elbow Baptist preachers in a few easy lessons. Today the backwoods swarm with chiropractors and in most states, they have been able to exert enough pressure upon the rural politicians to get themselves licensed. Any lout with strong hands and arms is perfectly equipped to become a chiropractor. No education beyond the elements is necessary. The whole art and mystery may be imparted in a few months, and the graduate is then free to practice upon God's images. The takings are often high, and so the profession has attracted thousands of recruits—retired baseball players, plumbers, truck drivers, longshoremen, bogus dentists, dubious preachers, village school superintendents. Now and then a quack doctor of some other school—say homeopathy—plunges into it. Hundreds of promising students come from the intellectual ranks of hospital orderlies.

In certain states, efforts have been made, sometimes by the medical fraternity, to make the practice of chiropractic unlawful. I am glad to be able to report that practically all of them have failed. Why should it be prohibited? I believe that every free-born man has a clear right, when he is ill, to seek any sort of treatment that he yearns for. If his mental processes are of such a character that the theory of chiropractic seems plausible to him, then he should be permitted to try chiropractic. And if it be granted that he has a right to do so, then it follows clearly that any stevedore privy to the technique of chiropractic has a right to treat him. To preach any contrary doctrine is to advocate despotism and slavery. The arguments for such despotism are all full of holes and especially those that come from medical men who have been bitten by the public hygiene madness, i.e. by the messianic delusion. Such fanatics infest every health department in the land. They assume glibly that the whole aim of civilization is to cut down the death rate and to attain that end they are willing to make a sacrifice of everything else imaginable including their own sense of humor. There is, as a matter of fact, not the slightest reason to believe that cutting down the death rate in itself is of much benefit to the human race. A people with an annual rate of 40 a thousand might still produce many Huxleys and Darwins, and one with a rate of but 8 or 9 might produce nothing but Coolidges and Billy Sundays. The former probability, in truth, is greater than the latter, for a low rate does not necessarily mean that more superior individuals are surviving; it may mean only that more of the inferior are surviving, and that the next generation will be burdened by their get.

Such quackeries as Christian Science, osteopathy and chiropractic work against the false humanitarianism of the hygienists and to excellent effect. They suck in the botched and help them on to bliss eternal. When these botched fall into the hands of competent medical men, they are very likely to be patched up and turned loose upon the world, to beget their kind. But massaged along the backbone to cure their lues, they quickly pass into the last stages, and so their pathogenic heritage perishes with them. What is too often forgotten is that nature obviously intends the botched to die, and that every interference with that benign process is full of dangers. Moreover, it is like birth control, profoundly immoral. The chiropractors are innocent in both departments. That their labors tend to propagate epidemics and so menace the lives of all of this, as is alleged by their medical opponents—this I doubt. The fact is that most infectious diseases of any seriousness throw out such alarming symptoms and so quickly that no sane chiropractor is likely to monkey with them. Seeing his patient break out in pustules or choking or falling into a stupor, he takes to the woods at once and leaves the business to the nearest medical men. His trade is mainly with ambulant patients; they must come to his studio for treatment. Most of them have lingering diseases; they tour all the neighborhood doctors before they reach him. His treatment, being essentially nonsensical, is in accord with the divine plan. It is seldom, perhaps, that he actually kills a patient, but at all events he keeps many a worthy soul from getting well.

Thus the multiplication of chiropractors in the Republic gives me a great deal of pleasure. It is agreeable to see so many morons getting slaughtered, and it is equally agreeable to see so many other morons getting rich. The art and mystery of scientific medicine, for a decade or more past, has been closed to all save the sons of wealthy men. It takes a small fortune to go through a class A medical college and by the time the graduate is able to make a living for himself, he is entering upon middle age, and is commonly so disillusioned that he is unfit for practice. Worse, his fees for looking at tongues and feeling pulses tend to be cruelly high. His predecessors charged 50 cents and threw in the pills; his own charges approach those of divorce lawyers, consulting engineers, and the higher hetaerrae.

Even general practice, in our great Babylons, has become a sort of specialty, with corresponding emoluments. But the chiropractor, having no such investment in his training, can afford to work for more humane wages, and so he is getting more and more of the trade. Six weeks after he leaves his job at the filling station or abandons the steering wheel of his motor truck, he knows all the anatomy and physiology that he will ever learn in this world. Six weeks more and he is adept at all the half-Nelsons and left hooks that constitute the essence of chiropractic therapy. Soon afterward, having taken postgraduate courses in advertising, salesmanship and mental mastery, he is ready for the practice. A sufficiency of patients, it appears, is always ready too. I hear no complaint from chiropractors of bad business. New ones are being turned out at a dizzy rate, but they all seem to find the pickings easy. Some time ago I heard of a chiropractor who, having once been a cornet player, had abandoned chiropractic in despair and gone back to cornet playing. But investigation showed that he was really not a chiropractor at all but an osteopath. The osteopaths, I am sure, are finding this new competition serious and unpleasant. As I have said, it was their Hippocrates, the late Dr. Still, who invented all the thrusts, lunges, yanks, hooks and bounces that the lowly chiropractors now employ with such vast effect, and for years the osteopath had a monopoly of them. But when they began to go scientific and ambitious, their course of training was lengthened until it took all sorts of tricks and dodges, borrowed from the regular doctors, or res-urrection men, including the plucking of tonsils, adenoids and appendices, the use of the stomach-pump and even some of the legerdemain of psychiatry. They now harry their students furiously and turn them out ready for anything from growing hair on a bald head to frying a patient with x-rays. All this new striving, of course, quickly brought its inevitable penalties. The os-teopath graduate, having sweated so long, was no longer willing to take a case of sarcoma for two dollars and in consequence he lost patients. Worse, very few aspirants could make the grade. The essence of osteopathy itself could be grasped by any lively farmhand or night watch-man in a few weeks, but the borrowed magic baffled him. Confronted by the phenomenon of gastrulation, or by the curious behavior of heart muscle, or by any of the curious theories of immunity, he commonly took refuge, like his brother of the orthodox faculty, in a gulp of laboratory alcohol, or fled the premises altogether. Thus he was lost to osteopathic science and the chiro-practors took him in; nay, they welcomed him. He was their meat. Borrowing that primitive part of osteopathy that was comprehensible to the meanest understanding, they threw the rest overboard at the same time denounc-ing it as a sorcery invented by the Medical Trust. Thus they gathered in the garage mechanics, ash-men and de-cayed welterweights, and the land began to fill with their graduates. Now there is a chiropractor at every crossroads, and in such sinks of imbecility as Los Angeles, they are as thick as bootleggers.

I repeat that it eases and soothes me to see them so prosperous, for they counteract the evil work of the so-called science of public hygiene, which now seeks to make morons immortal. If a man, being ill of a pus appendix, resorts to a shaved and fumigated longshoreman to have it disposed of and submits willingly to a treatment involving balancing him on McBurney's spot and playing on his vertebrae as on a concertina, then I am willing, for one, to believe that he is badly wanted in Heaven. And if that same man, having achieved lawfully a lovely babe, hires a blacksmith to cure its diphtheria by pulling its neck, then I do not resist the divine will that there shall be one less radio fan in 1967. In such matters, I am convinced the laws of nature are far better guides than the fiats and machinations of the medical busybodies who now try to run us. If the latter gentlemen had their way, death, save at the hands of hangmen, Prohibition agents and other legalized assassins, would be abolished altogether, and so that present differential in favor of the enlightened would disappear. I can't convince myself that would be of any good to the world. On the contrary, it seems to me that the current coddling of the half-witted should be stopped before it goes too far—if, indeed, it has not gone too far already. To that end, nothing operates more cheaply and effectively than the prosperity of quacks. Every time a bottle of cancer specific goes through the mails, Homo americanus is improved to that extent. And every time a chiropractor spits on his hands and proceeds to treat a gastric ulcer by stretching the backbone, the same high end is achieved.

But chiropractic, of course, is not perfect. It has superb potentialities, but only too often they are not converted into concrete cadavers. The hygienists rescue many of its foreordained customers, and, turning them over to agents of the Medical Trust, maintained at the public expense, get them cured. Moreover, chiropractic itself is not certainly fat: even an Iowan with diabetes may survive its embraces. Yet worse, I have a suspicion that it sometimes actually cures. For all I know (or any orthodox pathologist seems to know), it *may* be true that certain malaises are caused by the pressure of vagrom vertebrae upon the spinal nerves. And it *may* be true that a hearty ex-boilermaker, by a vigorous yanking and kneading, may be able to relieve that pressure. What is needed is a scientific inquiry into the matter, under rigid test conditions, by a committee of men learned in the architecture and plumbing of the body, and of a high and incorruptible sagacity. Let a thousand patients be selected, let a gang of selected chiropractors examine their backbones and determine what is the matter with them, and then let these diagnoses be checked up by the exact methods of scientific medicine. Then let the same chiropractors essay to cure the patients whose maladies have been determined. My guess is that the chiropractors' errors in diagnosis will run at least 95% and that their failures in treatment will push 99%. But I am willing to be convinced.

Where is such a committee to be found? I undertake to nominate it at ten minutes' notice. The land swarms with men competent in anatomy and pathology, and yet not engaged as doctors. There are hundreds of roomy and well-heated hospitals, with endless clinical material. I offer to supply the committee with cigars and music during the test. I offer, further, to supply both the committee and the chiropractors with sound pre-war wet goods. I offer, finally, to give a bawdy banquet to the whole Medical Trust, at the conclusion of the proceedings.

—H.L. Mencken

5

At Your Own Risk:
The Case against Chiropractic **(1969)**

In 1969, Ralph Lee Smith's book *At Your Own Risk: The Case Against Chiropractic* [1] provided a detailed look at chiropractic's shortcomings. The book's cover carried a bold statement by then-Chief Medical Examiner of New York City, Dr. Milton Helpern: "The teachers, research workers and practitioners of medicine reject the so-called principle on which chiropractic is based and correctly and bluntly label it a fraud and a hoax on the human race."

Despite this scorching indictment—and the underlying facts on which it was based—the number of licensed chiropractors in the United States has risen from about 23,000 at that time to between 55,000 and 70,000 in 2001, according to the American Chiropractic Association (ACA) Web site, and some 4,000 students graduate from chiropractic colleges each year. Furthermore, chiropractors are licensed in all 50 states, whereas in 1969 Louisiana and Mississippi still refused to grant them licenses.

Lousiana's refusal had been upheld by the U.S Supreme Court, which ruled that states could deny such license if they desired and had the right to insist on uniform, specific educational standards for entrance into the healing arts. During the trial, there was disagreement about whether chiropractors should engage in diagnosis. There was evidence that the chiropractic theory of subluxation was unscientific and that many chiropractors engaged in unscientific practices. The court did not address whether chiropractic theory was, in fact, scientific, but only that the chiropractic theory of a single cause and treatment of disease was wrong [2].

43

Smith described the Supreme Court's decision this way:

> The state has a right to insist on uniform educational and scientific standards for entering the healing arts. This test, which is an elementary one, is nevertheless one that chiropractic cannot meet because its beliefs and practices are scientifically false [1].

Louisiana's legislature and public health officials had stubbornly and steadfastly pointed out that "the emperor had no clothes." The only proper course that other states should have taken was to follow Louisiana's precept that health care laws should accord with science. This would have meant the end of the Iowa grocer's dream. Unfortunately, that did not happen. With persistent lobbying, licensing laws were enacted in Mississippi in 1973 and Louisiana in 1974 [3].

Chiropractic has indeed made many political gains in the past 30 years, as have many other "alternative" health care practices. One of the major gains was Congress's inclusion of chiropractic in the Medicare system despite a negative report by then-Secretary of the Department of Health, Education, and Welfare (HEW) Wilbur J. Cohen. The 1968 HEW report concluded:

> 1. There is a body of basic scientific knowledge related to health, disease and health care. Chiropractic practitioners ignore or take exception to much of this knowledge despite the fact that they have not undertaken adequate scientific research.
>
> 2. There is no valid evidence that subluxation, if it exists, is a significant factor in disease processes. Therefore, the broad application to health care of a diagnostic procedure such as spinal analysis and a treatment analysis such as spinal adjustment is not justified.
>
> 3. The inadequacies of chiropractic education, coupled with the theory that de-emphasizes proven causative factors in disease processes, proven methods of treatment and differential diagnosis, make it unlikely

that a chiropractor can make an adequate diagnosis and know the appropriate treatment, and subsequently provide the indicated treatment or refer the patient. Lack of these capabilities in independent practitioners is undesirable because appropriate treatment could be delayed or prevented entirely; appropriate treatment might be interrupted or stopped completely; the treatment offered could be contraindicated; all treatments have some risk involved with their administration and inappropriate treatment exposes the patient to this risk unnecessarily.

4. Manipulation (including chiropractic manipulation) may be a valuable technique for relief of pain due to loss of mobility of joints. Research in this area is inadequate; therefore, it is suggested that research based upon a scientific method be undertaken with respect to manipulation [4].

The HEW report recommended:

Chiropractic theory and practice are not based upon the body of basic knowledge related to health, disease and health care which has been widely accepted by the scientific community. Moreover, irrespective of its theory, the scope and quality of chiropractic education do not prepare the practitioner to make an adequate diagnosis and provide appropriate treatment. Therefore, it is recommended that chiropractic service not be covered in the Medicare program [4].

Despite these conclusions, which basically hold true today, Congress amended the Medicare law to include limited chiropractic coverage, as follows:

A chiropractor who is licensed as such by the state (or in a state which does not license chiropractors as such, is legally authorized to perform the services of a chiropractor in the jurisdiction in which he performs such services) and who meets uniform, minimum standards promulgated by the secretary . . . with respect to treatment by means of manual manipulation of the spine (to correct a subluxation demonstrated by x-ray to exist), which he is legally authorized to perform by the state or jurisdiction by which such treatment is provided.

The key provision of this enactment were the words to *"correct a subluxation demonstrated by x-ray to exist."* The "subluxations" postulated by chiropractic theory have never been demonstrated by x-ray or by any other imaging technique, including the newest computed tomography scans and magnetic resonance imaging studies—or for that matter, by any other means such as surgery or autopsy. Many chiropractors now describe subluxations as dynamic or functional spinal lesions rather than entities visible by x-ray [5].

The x-ray provision should have eliminated chiropractors from receiving Medicare payments, but since no one challenged it, Congress itself inadvertently became part of the chiropractic hoax. In 1997, Congress eliminated the x-ray requirement as of January 1, 2000.

Chiropractic's Alleged Scope

The HEW report noted that chiropractors claimed to treat nearly every type of illness [4]. The *Textbook of Office Procedures and Practice Building for the Chiropractic Profession* listed 92 illnesses that chiropractors treated and the average number of adjustments needed for each one. As Figure 1 notes, the average number of recommended adjustments ranged from 22.3 for appendicitis to 84.1 for jaundice. Ralph Lee Smith quipped that deafness then required 33.2 adjustments to cure, whereas it only took D.D. Palmer one, in his original chiropractic case.

In addition, in a survey reported in 1963 by the ACA [4], 7% of chiropractors said they treated cancer. (I recall a case of a spinal bone cancer I discovered in a patient being treated by a chiropractor. When I called the chiropractor to inform him

Condition	Average Number of Adjustments
Acne	28.2
Angina Pectoris	32.1
Appendicitis	22.3
Arthritis	49.0
Deafness	33.2
Diabetes	51.3
Epilepsy	76.1
Eye Disorders	42.5
Goiter	43.3
Heart Disorders	36.8
Hemorrhoids	50.9
High Blood Pressure	32.1
Jaundice	84.1
Kidney Disorders	43.2
Menstrual Disorders	33.1
Nephritis	34.1
Obesity	47.3
Palsy	63.7
Parkinson's Disease	57.6
Pneumonia	28.6
Polio, Acute	34.6
Polio, Chronic	51.3
Prostate Trouble	42.9
Rheumatic Fever	52.2
Ulcers	46.2

Figure 1. Average number of chiropractic adjustments reported for 25 of the "most frequent 100 conditions" seen in about 250,000 patients who received more than 10 million adjustments. Source: Parker JW. *Textbook of Office Procedures and Practice Building for the Chiropractic Profession*, Editions 1–4. Fort Worth, TX: Parker Chiropractic Research Foundation, 1964–1975.

NOTE: The book does not indicate how the diagnoses were made or how the data were obtained.

of the diagnosis and asked why he was manipulating the affected bones, he replied, "So what, you can't do anything about
cancer either.")

State licensing laws do little to restrict the scope of
chiropractic practice because they do not infringe on the
chiropractic philosophy or approach to health and disease. If
chiropractors limited themselves to treating conditions that truly
have a spinal cause, they would treat none of the conditions
listed in Figure 1. It is hard to imagine how chiropractors who
persuade patients to rely on spinal manipulation for appendicitis,
rheumatic fever, diabetes, heart disease, or any other serious
medically treatable disease could avoid being sued into oblivion.
Fortunately, the percentage of chiropractors willing to do such
treatment is much lower today than it was in the 1960s.

Revealing Personal Experiences

To prepare for the writing of *At Your Own Risk*, Smith decided
to visit chiropractic clinics as a patient. First, he had a thorough
cardiac and spinal evaluation at a major medical center, where
his physical condition was judged to be normal. Then he visited
the Palmer College of Chiropractic Clinic where he reported
having the typical symptoms of sciatic pain due to a ruptured
disk. Palmer College was nationally recognized at that time as a
"straight" school, meaning that its students were taught to practice strictly according to the Palmer belief in "subluxations"
and "adjustments," whereas the "mixers" included modalities
such as vitamins, minerals, and other nutritional methods.

At Palmer, Smith promptly underwent a "full spine x-
ray, front and side," which confirmed the chiropractor's "physical findings of three "subluxations," one in the fifth lumbar,
two in the ninth thoracic vertebra and three in the odontoid process in the neck." The perfunctory treatment consisted of a series of sudden thrusts and twists of his back, which caused him
soreness for about 2 weeks. This was followed by manipulation
of his neck by rolling his head and twisting his neck repeatedly

until a snap was heard and the "adjustment" was pronounced as successful. When Smith asked what disease he was suffering, he was told that (a) chiropractors do not diagnose or identify illness, (b) they simply remove the cause in the spine, and (c) he should continue to be adjusted by his local chiropractor to prevent recurrence.

Then Smith visited the clinic at the National College of Chiropractic, where he presented himself with the typical symptoms of coronary artery disease of a year's duration. After describing his symptoms of chest pain, which his cardiologist had told him were classic, he was seen by the assistant director of the hospital, who did not question him about his symptoms but proceeded to examine his neck and back. This chiropractor then announced that he had found "subluxations" at the fifth thoracic vertebra and proceeded to make the "adjustments." When a "pop" was heard, he manipulated Smith's neck and "jerked it to the left and to the right getting a good sharp pop each time." This college was noted for training "mixers," yet Smith received only the standard manipulative treatment for what should have been diagnosed as a heart condition.

Although what Smith reported sounds ludicrous as well as unscientific, most chiropractic licensing laws are so loosely worded and/or enforced that chiropractors can pretend that nearly all health problems are within their scope and that they even provide "complete health care." That chiropractors are still practicing this incredible hoax was exposed in a "20/20" ABC television program, by *Consumer Reports,* and by various advertisements discussed elsewhere in this book.

Smith's experience reminds me of the story of a man in his 40s, who would have been my father-in-law. Suffering from pain in his chest, left arm, and shoulder, he visited a chiropractor who gave him a "good working over," which the man said left him very tired. That night—as my wife has told me—the pain became worse and he died of a massive heart attack, leaving his wife and three young children to fend for themselves.

Such a failure to make a proper medical diagnosis of coronary artery disease and begin proper treatment was inexcusable then but would be even more so today because much more can now be done for heart attacks. We have balloon angioplasty, bypass surgery, and clot busters to dissolve the clots that cause the attacks, as well as preventive measures of proper lifestyle, exercise, low-fat diets, treatments for high blood pressure, and medications for high cholesterol. Clearly the clinical diagnosis of these conditions requires scientific medical knowledge and experience that is not available at chiropractic clinics. Heart attacks and their treatment certainly have nothing whatsoever to do with the spinal column or manipulative treatment of anything.

Smith described chiropractic marketing techniques taught 30 years ago, some of which are still in use today. One technique was to frighten people away from scientific treatment by alleging that its methods are deadly but chiropractic is a safe, natural treatment that does not use dangerous drugs or surgery. Smith also noted how chiropractors had the audacity to warn that scientific medicine dealt only with the "symptoms of disease" while chiropractors attack and eliminate the "true cause." [1] Exactly the opposite is true. This can be verified by examining any medical textbook in which the causes of disease are defined in scientific terms along with the symptoms, physical findings, laboratory and other tests, and detailed treatment. Spinal manipulation is intended to relieve pain, which is a symptom.

One chiropractor called me after reading several of my articles in my medical column on chiropractic to complain that I was bashing only chiropractors and not medical doctors and then asked why. I frankly answered that I thought chiropractic was the greatest hoax ever perpetrated on the American public. I then asked him—considering chiropractic objections to the use of antibiotics—whether he would use penicillin if he developed pneumonia. He replied that he would only use it if he were "sick enough." I then asked whether he realized that if the toxin produced by the bacterial infection had overwhelmed his system, penicillin would no longer be effective and he might die. This ended the conversation.

After visiting chiropractic clinics, Smith decided to attend a course in practice-building. Posing as a chiropractor, he was amazed at the blatant manner in which chiropractors built their practice. One lecture advised chiropractors to "dig for chronicity" by asking questions suggesting that the patient's symptoms represent a flareup of a chronic condition. Then the patient could be persuaded that the condition calls for a series of treatments and that cure might take a long time.

Attendees were also advised to push x-rays but not to use the word x-ray because this might frighten people. Instead, they were advised to say, "Let's take a few pictures." Medical science has discovered that excess x-ray exposure can cause harmful effects, including cancers, and that full-spine films are certainly not necessary and lack the detail required for accurate x-ray diagnosis. Medical science sees no need for full-length spinal x-rays, which can also influence the reproductive organs and result in birth defects. Nevertheless, the members of the well-attended conference were told that "x-rays should be given to most patients that come into the office and they should be the big 14 x 36 photos, if for no other reason than psychological."

The sum and substance of this experience left the impression with Smith that chiropractors were being taught to be smooth con artists, educated in the art of luring unsuspecting patients into a lifetime of chiropractic care. From the advertisements that I have seen as a columnist, little has changed during the past 30 years.

Shortly after the *Hartford Courant* (of Connecticut) ran a story on my legislative attempts to ban the use of chiropractic on children and cervical spine manipulation on anybody, I received a phone call from a medical secretary who was afraid to give her name but said she just had to tell me about her experience.

She stated that in response to an advertisement for employment, she sought a position in the office of a local chiropractor. She noted that the office appeared neat, well equipped with an x-ray machine and treatment table, and quite professional overall. She was hired and was quite satisfied with her work until she realized that the chiropractor recommended that all patients undergo the same x-ray examination and spinal manipulations regardless of their complaints and diagnosis. Furthermore, the chiropractor began to insist that she and her co-worker undergo neck "adjustments" so that they would stay strong and healthy and that they also bring family members in for similar treatments.

Her co-worker, fearful for her job, complied by submitting to neck "adjustments" and brought in other members of her family, but this secretary refused. One day, while she was sitting at her desk working, the chiropractor suddenly came up from behind, seized her by the neck and began twisting it. She struggled free and fled the office, never to return. She felt that she had to tell me this so that I would continue working for passage of my bill.

Anecdotes like this illustrate the tendency of "subluxation"-based chiropractors to urge virtually everyone they encounter to use their services. Whether this behavior is based on misguided belief, greed, or both makes little difference. There is no scientific evidence or plausible reason to believe that periodic "adjustments" make people healthier.

Smith concluded that licensing laws provide chiropractors with undeserved credibility:

> The public cannot be blamed for not realizing that chiropractic has no scientific foundation. This is the legislature's fault. People should be able to assume, and obviously do assume, that a state licensed "doctor" is practicing a valid, healing art [1].

Smith states that the public incorrectly assumes that the standards for measures taken by agencies such as the Food and Drug Administration, which oversees substantial provisions for the safety and effectiveness of drugs and medical technologies, are equally applied to chiropractic. He quotes Dr. Ralph E. Snyder, then-president and dean of New York Medical College, who said:

It is an incredible anachronism that in an age when this nation leads the world in many areas of scientific endeavor, New York State should be asked to place its seal of approval on a group of persons claiming to be practitioners who are largely ignorant of the accepted and proven science of health and disease [1].

Smith's book ends by discussing the idea that chiropractic colleges could be converted into medical schools. Smith did not believe this would be possible. Instead, he suggested three principles for seeking a political solution to the chiropractic problem:

1. Health-related laws that pay no attention to science show a deep failure on the part of legislators to fulfill their responsibility to their constituents and should be abolished.

2. Anyone claiming to have a valid treatment for human illness should be required to show his validity before the Bar of Science before receiving a state license to use it on the sick.

3. The correct way to deal with treatment methods that cannot or will not submit to the judgment of scientific research is not to limit and oversee them but to prohibit them. By abandoning all these precepts in the face of political pressures created by chiropractors, state legislators have created a state-supported medical superstition. The practice of chiropractic should therefore be prohibited and its personnel should be retrained to enter other professions [1].

If nothing else, Smith's revealing work provides proof for the French expression "*plus ca change, plus c'est la meme chose,*" which means the more things change, the more they remain the same—or even worse in 2001. The full text of *At Your Own Risk* is available on the Chirobase Web site at http://www.chirobase.org.

References

1. Smith RL. At Your Own Risk: The Case Against Chiropractic. New York: Pocket Books, 1969.
2. England vs Louisiana State Board of Medical Examiners (246 F Supp 993), cited by Monaghan WJ. No double standards for patient care. Journal of the American Medical Association 206:2191–2182, 1968.
3. Peterson D, Wiese G. Chiropractic: An Illustrated History. St. Louis: Mosby Year Book, 1995.
4. Cohen WJ. Independent Practitioners under Medicare: A Report to Congress. Washington, DC: Department of Health, Education, and Welfare, 1968.
5. Haldeman S, editor. Principles and Practice of Chiropractic, Second Edition. Norwalk, CT: Appleton & Lange, 1992.

6

The Views of
Consumer Reports (1975, 1994)

Consumer Reports (CR), which is highly respected for its independent no-nonsense evaluations of products and services, has published two comprehensive reports on chiropractic based on extensive investigations, one in 1975 and the other in 1994. Both point out the political gains made by chiropractic but deplore the lack of scientific evidence to back up many of its claims.

The 1975 report, titled "Chiropractors: Healers or Quacks," had two parts, titled, "The 80 Year War with Science" and "Can They Help? Do They Harm?" Part I explained in detail why chiropractic theory was wrong, laid bare the shortcomings of chiropractic education, and blasted the unethical practice-building strategies that were rampant at that time. Part II acknowledged that spinal manipulation might relieve back pain caused by restricted spinal joint mobility, but it warned that chiropractors falsely claimed to do much more, tended to take too many x-ray films, and sometimes injured patients with manipulations. The bottom-line advice was: "If you were planning to see a chiropractor, we think you would be safer to reconsider."

The 1994 report noted that "in recent years, several academic chiropractors have tried to correct such abuses and bring their profession into the scientific mainstream. . . . But in many cases, the problems we identified two decades ago still exist." The report charitably noted that D.D. Palmer's subluxation theory—when proposed in 1895—might have been a "reasonable stab at understanding the mysteries of health and disease" but should have been abandoned by now.

The centerpiece of the report was a survey sent to 456 chiropractors chosen randomly from an American Chiropractic

Association (ACA) membership directory. To carry out this survey, *CR*'s reporter posed as a prospective patient moving to the chiropractor's area with a husband, three young children, and a mother-in-law. About 60% of the chiropractors responded, many of them with printed literature and/or other information. The majority said that they focused on family health care. Nearly half the replies specifically mentioned that chiropractic can benefit children or included booklets with that implication. One chiropractor wrote, "Children are an essential part of my health outlook as they are (hopefully) the healthy adults of tomorrow." Another told how his 3-year-old son enjoys getting regular "adjustments." Another sent a long list of conditions "regularly treated" in his office, including allergies, depression, hypoglycemia, and prostate problems. It was clear from this that chiropractors, whether or not specifically allowed to by their licenses, claim that their scope is very broad.

If chiropractors would limit themselves to treating back pain and other musculoskeletal problems, they might win a broader measure of acceptance from medical doctors. However, many chiropractors want to do more. Louis Sportelli, DC, a former ACA board chairman, told *CR* that most people go to chiropractors initially for back and neck problems. Once they are in the office, he added, "practitioners educate them about the other conditions they can treat such as irritable bowel syndrome, dysfunctional gallbladder, functional forms of asthma and angina."

Some of the other key points in *CR*'s article, interspersed with my own comments, are described in the following.

The Well-Adjusted Child

The executive director of the Montreal Children's Hospital has appealed to pediatric hospitals throughout Canada to denounce chiropractic treatment of minors, which he considers "akin to child abuse." Yet chiropractors such as Jennifer and Palmer Peet claim in their textbook, *Chiropractic Pediatrics and Prenatal*

Reference Manual, "Thousands of infants and children die every week because they never receive chiropractic care." According to the Peets, infants should be checked for spinal misalignment and "subluxation" within hours of birth because the birth process can cause damage to the spine that may result in colic, impaired immunity, and even sudden infant death syndrome. This ludicrous claim is alive and well today, as described in Chapter 12 in this book, which discusses the treatment of headaches.

Dr. Jeffrey Young, an osteopathic physician who is board-certified in pediatrics, states flatly that these chiropractic claims have "absolutely no medical data to support them" or to justify chiropractic for epilepsy, asthma, bed-wetting, or learning disabilities, which are some of the many pediatric problems chiropractors claim they can treat.

Another troubling aspect of chiropractic that *CR* emphasizes is its traditional opposition to childhood immunizations. It was only in 1993 that the ACA officially abandoned its opposition. The New York Chiropractic College, however, has conducted seminars around the country questioning the value of immunizations, and 60% of chiropractors in their random sampling agreed with, or were ambivalent about, the college's statement, "There is no scientific proof that immunization prevents infectious disease." On the other hand, *CR* points out, chiropractic has failed to produce scientific evidence that it can prevent or cure any childhood disease.

Lifetime Patients

CR cites the continual "hard sell" efforts of chiropractic to establish lifetime patients, as Smith described in his book *At Your Own Risk* in 1969. *CR* mentions promoters like Alan Bernstein, president of the "Practice Builder," and David Singer, a Clearwater, Florida, chiropractor who sells an audiotape set called "How to Create Lifetime Patients." Promoting lifetime patients or maintenance care is a favorite strategy of practice-management firms. *CR* found some 50 such companies offering courses and literature to chiropractors on how to build their practices.

Some of the catch phrases recommended by these promotion consultants are "maintenance care"; "ensuring spinal health"; and for anyone questioning the need for lifetime care, "It is a choice you, yourself, must make, depending on how important your health is." The Peter Pan Potential, a California-based marketing company, advises, "Go to the children." Another suggestion is for chiropractors to get patients to sign up friends' children for free examinations.

However, Scott Haldeman, MD, DC, in his *Practice and Principles of Chiropractic* textbook, does admit, "There are no long term outcome trials on the value of preventive chiropractic care" to justify such maintenance care promotion.

Nutrition and Applied Kinesiology

Although nutrition has nothing to do with traditional chiropractic, the "mixers" use this as a means of broadening their activities. Since they are uneducated in the use of medicines and are not licensed to prescribe them, they resort to vitamins, minerals, and food to treat or prevent disease. The classic example of this was demonstrated on the "20/20" ABC television exposé in which a chiropractor advised a mother to have her child stop drinking milk to clear his ear infection and suggested that allergy to milk might be the cause of the infection. (It is difficult to see why this nonsensical chiropractic advice is not subject to lawsuits even if it is judged standard chiropractic care.)

In a 1991 survey, the National Board of Chiropractic Examiners (NBCE) found that 84% of responding chiropractors had used nutritional counseling therapy or supplementation within the previous 2 years and that 30% had used homeopathic remedies. (Homeopathic remedies are minute doses of various materials claimed to produce the same symptoms in healthy persons as the disease itself. Their theoretical basis is nonsensical, and they have no scentifically proven value.)

"Applied kinesiology," used by 37% of respondents to the NBCE survey, is based on the notion that every organ dysfunction is accompanied by special muscle weakness and that disease can be diagnosed by testing muscles after placing food or nutrient substances under the tongue.

Even more bizarre, I saw a 1-hour television program in which a Connecticut chiropractor demonstrated a diagnostic method called contact reflex analysis (CRA), which he described as an extension of applied kinesiology and acupuncture. He claimed that muscle-testing related to "reflex points" could be used to diagnose problems throughout the body.

To demonstrate, he asked the television hostess to extend one arm to the side while he touched the supposed "reflex points" and pushed down on her arm. He touched between her eyes to "test" the pituitary gland, on her neck for the thyroid, at her umbilicus for intestinal disease, and her chest for heart disease. When he tested her lower abdomen, her arm went down, which he attributed to "low salt" in the body. CRA is about as senseless as anything can be, but the chiropractor stated he has been using it with great success in his practice for 20 years.

Safety

Chiropractors say their methods are safer than surgery and drugs that have dangerous and toxic side effects. There is some truth in this because medical doctors often treat critically ill patients with drugs, all of which may have side effects. But the risk/benefit ratio is in favor of medical doctors. For example, a serious reaction to penicillin may happen once in 1 million uses, yet many lives are saved with the 999,999 other penicillin injections.

The companies that insure chiropractors for malpractice won't reveal how many claims they have received or paid out for patients who have suffered a stroke or paralysis after having their neck manipulated. The number is not large compared with the number of necks that have been manipulated. But whatever it is, it may only represent the tip of the iceberg because only a small fraction of injured patients file a lawsuit. Back manipulation can also produce serious injury. And when manipulation is done without good reason—as it often is—no complication is excusable.

In terms of safety, most people who consult chiropractors are x-rayed, which poses a danger of x-ray radiation, especially from the full-spinal type used to locate nonexistent "subluxations." These full-length x-rays do not provide sharp images, and the x-ray dosage required to produce them can increase the likelihood of birth defects in a patient's offspring.

Recommendations

The 1994 *CR* article states that "if you are thinking about going to a chiropractor for back pain, proceed with caution" and follow these guidelines:

- See your doctor first for the correct diagnosis of your problem.
- Remember that manipulation of the neck may be risky, especially if you take oral contraceptives or anticoagulant drugs, or if you have high blood pressure or other risk factors for stroke.
- Get a referral from a reliable source, such as the National Association for Chiropractic Medicine (NACM) in the United States or the Orthopractic Manipulation Society in Canada, or consider getting a referral to a physical therapist.
- Inquire by telephone about the nature of the chiropractor's approach.

CR recommended NACM and the Orthopractic Society because their members have abandoned the subluxation theory; do not try to treat children, infections, or other diseases; and limit their practice to the treatment of musculoskeletal problems (mostly back pain). Another way to locate clear-thinking chiropractors is the referral directory on the Chirobase.org Web site, which was not available when *CR* published its article.

7

Smart Money
Hits a Raw Nerve (1997)

The January 1997 issue of *Smart Money*, the *Wall Street Journal*'s magazine of personal finance and related matters, included an insightful article titled "Ten Things Your Chiropractor Won't Tell You." [1] The article was written by John Protos, who called me several times for information. This chapter lists the 10 points with additional comments from me.

1. "I've got more nutty theories than Oliver Stone."
While acknowledging that chiropractic techniques can be effective, Protos points out—in so many words—that chiropractic theory is still a hoax. He also notes that "some chiropractors believe that by manipulating ('adjusting') someone's back, they can treat almost any malady from arthritis and allergies to kidney failure and . . . hearing loss" and that "even those who don't explicitly claim that chiropractic is a cure-all often contend that their training enables them to diagnose every kind of ailment." (Oliver Stone directed the fictional movie *JFK* about the "conspiracy" to murder President John F. Kennedy.)

2. "My bill will be the real back-breaker."
Although people go to a chiropractor because they think chiropractors are cheaper, *Smart Money* notes that a study published in the *New England Journal of Medicine* in 1995 found that seeing a chiropractor for acute low back pain cost an average of $611 in rural areas and $783 in urban areas, whereas the average cost of seeing a primary-care medical doctor was $474 in rural areas and $508 in urban areas. These differences occurred

because the medical treatment typically involved two visits, but the rural chiropractors saw patients nine times and the urban ones saw them for 13 visits [2].

3. "Go elsewhere to be on the safe side."
Your chiropractor won't tell you to go elsewhere—to an osteopath or physiatrist (medical doctor who specializes in physical medicine) if you want manipulation alone or with other treatment. Medical and osteopathic physicians are better trained than chiropractors and offer a much wider range of treatments. In addition to (or instead of) manipulation, they can prescribe medications and physical therapy. They (or their surgical colleagues) can also cure some cases of ruptured disk, spinal tumor, or other causes of back pain.

4. "I could make things worse."
Smart Money describes the case of Tamara Joerns, a 27-year-old mother of three children in California who was paralyzed from the neck down from a stroke caused by a neck manipulation. Joerns sued the chiropractor, but the judge ruled that the chiropractor's manipulation did not amount to substandard care. In Chapter 6, I describe how a Connecticut woman won a $10 million malpractice award after a similar experience. The frequency of these cases is unknown, largely because chiropractic malpractice insurance companies keep their data secret. But they occur often enough to know that neck manipulation carries some degree of hazard.

5. "Your health insurer thinks I'm a slouch."
Although many chiropractors advertise that they "accept most health insurance plans," anyone contemplating treatment should check their coverage carefully. Insurance companies are not particularly fond of chiropractors. Although "insurance equality laws" in most states force companies to pay for certain chiropractic services, the coverage may be skimpy (e.g., partial payment and a limited number of visits), and about half of employers who self-insure don't include chiropractic coverage.

6. "We'll be seeing a lot of each other."
Smart Money asks, "How long should a sequence of visits to your chiropractor last?" The article cites chiropractic sources whose answers seem to be, "Forever." A pamphlet from the Garden State Chiropractic Society states, "It doesn't make sense to wait until a crisis occurs and do something about your health. By having your spine checked regularly—regardless of how you feel—you have taken a sensible step towards health maintenance." A prominent chiropractic practice-building firm has marketed audiotapes called "How to Create Lifetime Patients" and a videotape series called "How to Educate Patients for Life." These materials teach how to persuade patients to come regularly for check-ups and spinal "adjustments" that allegedly "work to remove the cause of problems before symptoms arise" and help people "feel better, increase endurance and reduce the risk of health problems." [3]

7. "We like 'em young."
Many chiropractors will start treatment on newborns, as documented in a television show I saw in which the chiropractor manipulated a newborn while saying, "As the twig is bent, so goes the tree." Not all chiropractors, however, agree that their treatment is suitable for children. *Smart Money* quotes Ron Slaughter, DC, of the National Association for Chiropractic Medicine, who says that (a) no child under 12 should ever be taken to a chiropractor unless recommended by a pediatrician; (b) chiropractic manipulations could interfere with a child's bone structure; and (3) the use of chiropractic manipulation for chronic ear infection, bed-wetting, and asthma is "bunk."

8. "The vitamins I'm prescribing will rejuvenate my wallet."
Many chiropractors who disparage the use of drugs eagerly sell vitamins and other dietary supplements to their patients, usually for at least twice their wholesale cost. Most of what they recommend has not been proven useful. *Smart Money* points out that patients who chose to take vitamins might probably find a retail or mail-order store that will charge less for it.

9. "X-rays are our best friend."

Some chiropractors run their x-rays like a profit center, passing the cost on to patients and insurance companies. One chiropractor interviewed for the article quipped, "They will x-ray people until they glow in the dark." Another stated, "Only 1 in 500 back x-rays will show something that was not expected." *Smart Money* mentions one insurance company that was suing a chiropractic group for fraudulently taking 700 x-rays on only 13 patients. Since the association between x-rays and cancer has been widely publicized, it amazes me that a patient would submit to more than 50 unnecessary spinal x-ray examinations.

10. "You probably will get better on your own."

Citing several reliable sources, *Smart Money* points out that two thirds of all patients with acute back pain will be pain-free after 6 weeks, with or without treatment, and that 90% of cases resolve on their own within 12 weeks.

When Jerome McAndrews, DC, an American Chiropractic Association spokesman, was asked why so many visits to the chiropractor were needed, he replied that the problem was really that of medical doctors because they treat only the symptoms of back pain—often with painkillers—whereas chiropractic techniques are more ambitious. "We go further in the analysis to address the causal problem," McAndrews claimed. "That usually requires more visits."

This is a major theme of chiropractic, that medical doctors only treat the symptoms, whereas they treat the cause of diseases. This claim is a pure and simple figment of chiropractic imagination. In fact, it is backwards. If anything, chiropractors only treat the symptoms of pain, whereas medical doctors often can treat the cause. This difference—based on medicine's scientific approach—has resulted in incredible advances in medical care throughout the world.

The March 1997 issue of *Smart Money* carried several letters to the editor that illustrate the typical chiropractic response to criticism:

• Jeffrey Wilder, DC, president of the Wisconsin Chiropractic Association, complained that the National Association for Chiropractic Medicine, quoted as critical of some chiropractic practices, particularly on children, is a radical splinter group with only a handful of members. He also cited the Agency of Health Care Policy and Research findings, analyzed in this book in Chapter 18, regarding the favorable report on spinal manipulation for low back pain.

• Another chiropractor cited the care of a patient who had multiple back injuries, which he claimed chiropractic treatment could have prevented.

• Charles A. Paine, DC, of Bridgewaters, New York, said that, "Quoting medical doctors on a story about chiropractic is like having inmates do a story about the police."

• David Pignatello, DC, of Seminole, Florida, said that an "eleventh thing a chiropractic won't tell you. . . . Subscribe to *Smart Money* magazine."

My letter, the only one from the scientific community, said:

> While many people feel they benefit from chiropractic treatment, there is no scientific proof that they are actually helped. The evidence is basically junk science based on anecdotal outcomes, for the most part. The theoretical chiropractic lesion, "the subluxation," pressing on a nerve, causing some disease, has never been demonstrated by operation, autopsy, x-ray, or any other means. In other words, chiropractic as defined does not exist.

References

1. Protos J. Ten things your chiropractor won't tell you. Smart Money, Jan 17, 1997, pp 107–109, 111, 113.
2. Carey TS and others. The outcomes and costs of care for acute low back pain among patients seen by primary care practitioners, chiropractors, and orthopedic surgeons. New England Journal of Medicine 333:913-917, 1995.
3. Singer D. Maintenance care [pamphlet]. Clearwater, FL: Expand Chiropractic Products, 1993.

8

The Lemmon/Matthau Takeoff

The comedy team of Jack Lemmon and Walter Matthau did a hilarious takeoff on chiropractic in their 1997 movie *Out to Sea*. Matthau played the part of a ne'er-do-well gambler and con man whose sister married Lemmon's character. The sister, whom Lemmon's character loved dearly, died, but he and Matthau's character remained close friends.

Lemmon played the part of a very ordinary fellow who had spent most of his life as a salesman employed at Gimbel's Department Store. He continued to carry a torch for his departed wife and could not show interest in other women. Matthau's character, a playboy bachelor, felt this was wrong and inveigled Lemmon's character to go on a cruise with him with arrangements he had conned from a friend. As part of the deal, unbeknown to Lemmon's character, he and Lemmon's character were supposed to act as dance hosts and entertain the ladies. Matthau's character, who knew nothing about dancing, feigned an injury to his leg and back, complaining to the ship's recreation manager that he had slipped on the wet dance floor.

Lemmon's character, recognizing the ruse and to get even with Matthau's character, proceeded to manhandle him with various twisting, leg thrusts, and manipulations. The acrobatics were obvious and drew more laughter than at any other point in the entire comedy, which had many funny moments.

As is the case with many comedies, a serious point was made. Comedy, whether intended it or not, is often the highest form of debunking a serious subject. Lemmon and Matthau depicted chiropractic as a joke. Here was a man feigning an injured leg and back, and the treatment he received made absolutely no sense. The audience recognized the situation as a hoax and enjoyed the scene immensely.

The two actors did not receive an Oscar for this performance, but they surely deserve accolades from the scientific medical community. Whether unwittingly or intended, their scene might make people think about the silliness of some of the things that chiropractors do.

Part III
My Own Investigations

9
The Crippling of
Linda Solsbury

Linda Solsbury is a former pediatric nurse and part-time ballet dancer whose encounter with chiropractic left her a completely helpless invalid[1]. She had sought chiropractic care to increase her dancing movements and agility but became quadriplegic from vertebral artery injury that occurred during neck manipulation by a chiropractor. The vertebral arteries, one on each side, thread through holes in the six upper vertebrae of the neck. Sudden neck rotation, particularly with the neck extended, can injure these arteries and interrupt the flow of blood to the base of the brain.

Vertebrobasilar strokes are rare and differ from the common type caused by blockage of a carotid artery, which affects only half of the body. In Solsbury's case, both arms and legs are paralyzed and she is unable to speak or swallow, yet she remains mentally clear. She can express her thoughts only by typing on a computer with one finger that still functions. Here is her story, as typed on her computer:

> To try and explain the impact—on every area of my life—is too overwhelming to even think about it. It's like setting up a giant set of dominoes and saying "let 'er rip." For the rest of my life—confined to a wheelchair—electric at that, to have any mobility—having only regained minimal use of my right hand. I have a feeding tube in my stomach, an indwelling catheter in my bladder (causing frequent infections requiring antibiotic therapy—often only—painful—intramuscular injections 1 x shift x 10 days is the only medication that

71

works—and when the bacteria build up my resistance to that ....???) using a portable computer to communicate—tedious is an understatement—time consuming—some can't see it, some are unable to read well—if at all—always aware of an undercurrent of impatience, the physical and occupational therapy. Needing complete care in bathing, dressing—needing to be mechanically transferred by a lift and sling—bed to chair and visa versa. Relying on someone to do everything for me—from watering my plants to making an envelope, to combing my hair. The indignity of no privacy with personal hygiene, i.e.—having someone else changing a tampon to being given enemas every other day to evacuate my bowels—and again—relying on another—whoever is assigned ... whether you like them or not ... whether they are good or marginal workers ... you get who you get. I will never again know the luxury of an uninterrupted night's sleep. I have 12 midnight tube feeding, 1 a.m., 4 a.m., 6:30 a.m. turns....because I need someone to change my position in bed. I have itches (endlessly) that are out of my reach. I like nights the most because sleep provides some escape. Evenings come in second best. I can occupy my mind more and days are my least favorite—because I am forced to deal more with the full impact of my limitations. The list goes on and on.....that doesn't begin to touch the emotional impact. That is—so far—beyond measurement.

People commonly believe a crisis tightens family bounds. In the short term, that may be true; in the long term, all too often, the reverse is true. My daughter cannot deal with this situation. She lives with her father and stepmother when not away at college. He makes it acceptable for her to feel justified in not coming. I rarely see her. It was tremendously painful to play the major role in her life to suddenly be on the outskirts of everything that happened. To "hear" about her prom, to "hear" about her graduation, to hear about her first love in vague comments—long after the fact, to not even hear about getting college acceptance letters. I would keep expecting her to "come to terms with things"—only to realize that this is the way it is going to be—"I have to come to terms with things." The man I was involved with took a position out of state. My closest friend moved out of state. My mother and I had such a fragile relationship to begin with—now it is almost nonexistent. My younger brother was the only family that visited on a regular basis; he died three years ago in the spring. My life is totally devoid of any type of affection. I spend every holiday alone. I always feel like a burden. I never feel attractive. I spend most of my time alone. I'm basically an introvert (sic) prior to my stroke—now I feel it's a forced isolation; like a monk in a monastery who took vows of silence and solitude.

I try to imagine ... what could be worse .. ? Well, I suppose I could be like this and live in a third world country .... that would be worse. I don't feel particularly sorry to hear if someone has a terminal illness. They have a way out. This is like a life sentence. No one can imagine what it is like to live this way ... they can try ... but there are too many facets, one outside—could never even consider. I hear how "lucky" I am to have my cognition. However wonderful of "others" to project their opinions (sic) ... when they can only have a very "one dimensional" view. I think "..you fools, ... you can't know .... it makes it harder." I see human nature from a vista few do.

For the most part, we are not so noble as we like to think.

My life is "imposed" on me in a physical sense and in an emotional sense—by some "challenging" my "will" to live (a sunset, a flower, a snowfall, touching, huh?..moxie (sic).. ??)—but the "will" to live—if you can really live—is this really living? It's existing ... I can tell you that. Am I supposed to "derive" something of worth from this? Is that a task I just haven't mastered yet? My life is today—and I imagine will always be— like walking a tightrope—everyday and seen as "deranged" or at the very least "maladapted" for speaking "my" truth? It's like the proverb: tell the truth and run. My way of seeing my life is wrong?? By others who don't awaken to this ... everyday.

It is like I had a bomb dropped in the middle of my life.

That does not begin to touch on how dehumanizing living in an institution is. Apart from the physical handicaps; it is like a mental bludgeoning to beat the psyche into a "herd mentality" until one's sense of self starts to fragment and shrivel.

As a nurse I could see family struggle to cope with tragedy; as much as I empathized, I still felt exempt. I no longer feel exempt.

The Chiropractor Responds

The six-person jury found Waterford, Connecticut, chiropractor Thomas P. Goulding's treatment to be the direct cause of the stroke. Despite this, and despite overwhelming evidence that such treatment has caused strokes in many other cases, Goulding denied all this in the following letter to the editor of the *Day*, a newspaper in New London, Connecticut, where the trial was held:

> The *Day* has, in recent weeks, published reports concerning my trial. I would like to set the record straight as your paper has only revealed the plaintiff's arguments.
>
> First, and most important, the chiropractic treatment did not cause Ms. Solsbury's stroke. The procedure described by the plaintiff's experts was never done in my

office in her several years of chiropractic care! Second, in response to Ms. Solsbury's column, I will remain in business and plan to remain serving the natural health care needs of our community for many years.

This was a tragic occurrence with a devastating residual to Ms. Solsbury, but the cause was not my treatment. This patient had numerous neurological complaints and symptoms from the early 1970s. At the time of this incident, she was post surgical and was self-medicating with prescription drugs when she had a stroke. One drug causes extreme vasospasm. She had a history of vascular disease.

People wonder why it took so long to get to trial. The major delay was the plaintiff's attorneys trying to obtain experts to say what they wanted and blame my treatment. They had to look far and wide, from Washington state to North Carolina to find their hired guns. One doctor had no college degree and had never seen the patient or read her medical records—but felt I was to blame. The other experts were very well credentialed and very well spoken professors and again blamed the chiropractic treatment. They had never been to a chiropractor; they had never seen a chiropractic adjustment performed; but they blamed the chiropractic treatment anyway.

You look long and hard enough, you can find someone to say whatever you want. In defending the case, we relied on the treating doctors' testimony. They agreed with me that the cause of this incident could not be determined. Originally, I was sued for two million five years ago. Over a year ago the plaintiff's attorney would have settled for $350,000, and they wanted my father's widow to kick in $100,000! All these figures were well beyond my reach. The plaintiff's attorney stated more than once his desire to "ruin my practice" and my wife's as well.

Mr. Swain (Solsbury's lawyer) had been very available to the press stating his altruism in not accepting a fee—there was no fee for him to accept; he will, though, have his expenses paid and the rest will go to the state. My expenses, however, ran well over $60,000! So over $100,000 was spent so that his client could get $500. Is this ethical? Mr. Swain also met with the sworn jury immediately after the verdict, which I have since learned is unacceptable in many courts.

The end product is that I must go bankrupt. I have no more resources to appeal this case. I do feel that I would win on an appeal, now knowing the tactics used against me. This has been a tremendous hardship on my family. It has been most difficult to be libeled in the press while deeply involved in this trial and at the same time have Mr. Swain making himself so available to describe his legal heroics on the plaintiff's behalf. All he has to show is $500 for his client. His expenses paid, a dramatic commercial for his law firm, and bankruptcy for me. Does this sound like justice?

The ultimate insult is that when a juror came forward and spoke to the judge about prejudice on the jury during deliberations, nothing was done. This has been a most terrible tragedy and my heart and prayers go out to Ms. Solsbury, and I can understand her wanting to blame someone. Attorneys, however, I cannot understand. Chiropractic has been helping to treat patients without drugs and without surgery for over 100 years. Chiropractic treatment does not cause strokes.

I would like to thank all the patients who have expressed their concerns and support. I have always treated my patients with kindness, concern and gentle treatment. I have had great respect for our legal process, but I am now much more sensitive to those wrongly accused.

Thomas P. Goulding, DC, Waterford

Other Views

Attorney Peter J. Bartinik, a member of the Board of Governors of the Connecticut Trial Lawyers' Association, sent the following letter to the editor of the *Day*:

> A jury had determined that Ms. Solsbury's injuries and horrendous disabilities were caused by the negligence of Thomas Goulding. What is appalling is that Dr. Goulding is unable to meet his professional responsibility because he failed to maintain what is commonly referred to as a professional liability insurance policy. What is appalling is that Ms. Solsbury will go uncompensated because Dr. Goulding had decided by not maintaining a professional insurance policy that the risk of his carelessness and negligence should be borne by his patients and not himself.

Solsbury, although hopelessly paralyzed, was able to salvage a bit of satisfaction by having an insurance bill passed that mandates malpractice insurance coverage for all Connecticut chiropractors and even appeared herself in dramatic testimony before the state legislature. She received national recognition for her work on the "Evening News with Connie Chung."

As for the proof that chiropractic neck manipulation has caused similar strokes, this was well documented during the trial by reports from the Mayo Clinic and from J. Donald Eastman, MD, of the Southern Illinois Medical School, who referred to 25 cases. A report by neurosurgeon Thomas Mehalic, MD, called chiropractic a "cultist mechanotherapy."

Solsbury herself described her stroke to me. Her first symptoms occurred during manipulation of her neck to improve her dancing. She became faint and sweaty, and that afternoon her speech became slurred and she experienced weakness in her legs. She was hospitalized at Lawrence and Memorial Hospital in intensive care. Here she had a convulsion and lapsed into coma from her stroke. She required a tracheostomy and respiratory resuscitation to save her life. I reported this incident in an article to our local *New Britain Herald* newspaper.

A local chiropractor, Edward F. Hartney, a frequent advertiser in the *Herald*, objected to what I said. In a letter to the editor, he stated:

> Publishing Dr. Chotkowski's response to the *Herald* article on the state's malpractice insurance laws was irresponsible on the *Herald*'s behalf. In fact, Chotkowski did not respond to the subject matter discussed and used the *Herald* to express one of his personal opinions. This patient's plight is horrible and I feel heartsick for her and her family. When and if a doctor is truly negligent, he or she must be held accountable. No concerned health care provider would treat a patient unless that person was protected in every way. Although the jury found on her behalf, I find it difficult to believe that a vertebral artery could experience a dissecting tear in a healthy young person. A chiropractic manipulative procedure is a gentle act based on the scientific principles of anatomy, physiology and the latest research in biomechanics.
>
> Chiropractic care is safe, efficient and cost effective. Over 10 million Americans visit doctors of chiropractic each year.
>
> Chiropractic care will prevail and become part of the new health plan because of public demand.

After reading this letter, Solsbury wrote the following letter directly to Hartney:

> My purpose in writing is to dissuade the opinions you stated in your Letter to the Editor of the *New Britain Herald*, September 24, 1993. With all due respect, I find your letter more in keeping with irresponsible use of the newspaper media. I hope the enclosed information causes you to reconsider your position.
>
> "Young and healthy" had nothing whatsoever to do with my injury. Improperly executed manipulation did.

Young and healthy was the reason I did not succumb; rather, was gravely ill, on life support and in ICU for several weeks.

I doubt that I was any different from a patient you might see in your practice. Five years of chiropractic treatment at various intervals, very attuned to the body, very open to alternative health care as a means to insure good health, avoid medications—risk free ... I thought
...

Those are two key words, Dr. Hartney. Chiropractic care is no more risk-free than conventional medicine. To imply that it is, in 1993, is very reckless. You are clearly not informed on what has been increasingly in medical and chiropractic literature for well over a decade. By lack of acknowledging this, you are denying your patients informed consent. It would be wise, if you expect to maintain patient confidence, to rethink your position on this matter. Public awareness of this danger is increasing. The results will be your clients going to chiropractors who will caution honestly.

In reference to chiropractic strokes, Solsbury included with the letter to Hartney a list of reports by experts such as Dr. Singer, chief of pediatric neurology at Cambridge Hospital, a teaching hospital for Harvard Medical School; Dr. Simon, head of neurosurgery at University of Connecticut Medical Center, a teaching hospital; and Dr. White, neuroradiologist, also at University of Connecticut Medical Center. These doctors were able to use angiography to demonstrate blood clots in torn vertebral and basilar arteries in patients who had suffered a stroke following chiropractic neck manipulation.

Further Observations

What can we conclude from this case, based on obvious facts? The following conclusions seem fair, based on the facts.

- Chiropractors either are ignorant of the hazards of neck manipulation or refuse to admit to the dangers and insist on continuing this practice.
- The risk/benefit of chiropractic neck manipulation makes this form of treatment prohibitive. Cervical spinal manipulation is a sometimes-lethal procedure for which there is no scientifically proven purpose.
- It is clear that patients are not being appropriately informed of the dangers of neck twisting. The exact incidence of similar strokes is unknown but appears to be considerable.
- This practice should be banned by licensure. (Through my representative, a bill was introduced to the Connecticut legislature, but this was trashed without a hearing by the Public Health Committee, whose chairman, Senator George Guenther, is a naturopath who believes that a chiropractor cured his polio when he was younger. Banning the procedure will not be easy.)

The journal *Stroke* has published additional evidence of the relationship between chiropractic care and the incidence of vertebrovascular accidents (VBAs) in nonelderly adults. Using hospital and insurance records, Canadian researchers compared VBA patients with similar patients who had been hospitalized for other problems. The data showed that VBA patients younger than 45 years were five times more likely than the others to have visited a chiropractor within a week of the VBA and to have had three or more visits with neck manipulations [2]. An accompanying editorial states that data correspond to an incidence of 1.3 cases of vertebral artery dissection or blockage per 100,000 individuals receiving chiropractic neck manipulation.

Cases like that of Linda Solsbury will continue to occur until the chiropractic neck-twisting practice that caused her tragedy is abolished, either by an act of the legislature, by prohibitive malpractice lawsuits, or by a voluntary chiropractic realization and resignation to scientific fact.

It is incredible that some chiropractors refuse to admit neck manipulation can cause strokes and death by injuring the vertebrobasilar artery system that supplies blood to the brain.

References

1. Personal communication and documentation from Linda Solsbury, 1997.
2. Rotherwell DM and others. Chiropractic manipulation and stroke. Stroke 32:1054-1060, 2001.

10

Visits to Two
Chiropractic Colleges

America's 125 medical schools are graduating about 15,000 physicians a year who will practice science-based medicine. Chiropractic's 16 colleges are producing about 4,000 graduates, most of whom will practice unscientifically. I find these relative numbers alarming.

To learn more about chiropractic education, I decided to visit a chiropractic college. I first called the American Chiropractic Association for information about such a visitation. I said that I was a medical journalist writing a weekly medical column and book in my retirement. They were most cooperative and arranged for a guided tour and an interview with the dean of New York Chiropractic College in Seneca, New York.

The tour guide was a young lady who was well versed in chiropractic philosophy, which she explained to a group of about 10 visitors, most of whom appeared to be prospective students. I asked several questions that the guide had some difficulty in answering. She referred me to the dean, whom I later interviewed.

New York Chiropractic College is located in the former Eisenhower College. The buildings are impressive, glitzy, alabaster structures surrounded by finely manicured, expansive lawns that would put to shame the medical school campuses of Yale (my alma mater) or Harvard. At the time of my visit (1997), the school had some 900 students and graduated about 300 chiropractors each year. Tuition was $4,170 each trimester, of which there were 10, for a total of $41,700 for 4 years. However, it is possible to complete chiropractic school in 3 years.

I saw 15 classrooms and laboratories, an ample number of x-ray film viewing boxes, and some strange looking examining tables designed for spinal manipulations and "adjustments." I noticed five medical doctors' names on the faculty but saw no evidence of any research department or activity to which the guide referred. The library contained a number of standard medical texts in addition to chiropractic publications.

The president of the college gave me a large package of information about chiropractic and a book entitled *Principles and Practice of Chiropractic*, edited by Dr. Scott Haldeman, a third-generation chiropractor who acquired a medical degree and now practices neurology. Some chiropractors appear to regard this book as their "chiropractic bible." It was to me a 600-page failed effort to explain exactly what chiropractic is supposed to be. An insert classified chiropractic as one of 45 major "alternative healthcare methodalities."

During my meeting with the dean, I said: "I am a medical columnist and admit to a scientific bias. I believe that chiropractic is the biggest medical hoax ever perpetrated on the American public. Please give me any evidence to the contrary. For starters, of the 14,000 or so diseases afflicting mankind, name one which chiropractic has proved scientifically to benefit or cure."

"Oh," the dean replied, "we do not treat disease. We treat wellness. We keep people healthy with periodic spinal adjustments."

"But," I pursued, "chiropractic in over 100 years has failed to demonstrate what is supposedly being adjusted. Despite surgery, autopsy, and sophisticated imagery, no spinal vertebral subluxation has ever been seen or shown to press on a nerve, interfering with the passage of energy down that nerve, causing disease, as chiropractic claims."

"That is because a vertebral subluxation is not an anatomical lesion. It is a 'dynamic lesion.' We call it a DSL or FSL, a dynamic or functional spinal lesion. (These definitions were corroborated in Haldeman's textbook.)

At this point, after a series of similar questions and answers, I suggested to the dean that there was clearly no satisfactory evidence of such an entity as chiropractic as defined and that they should convert their college into a medical school and abandon this phony chiropractic theory.

It is not difficult to see how young people can easily be seduced into this field by becoming a "doctor" in a few shorter and less expensive years. The college aura; the academic-appearing catalog; and the neat, shiny, scientific-looking classrooms certainly must be enticing.

My Report Draws Comments

I shared the details of this visit with my medical colleagues in a letter to the editor of *Connecticut Medicine* in the June 1997 issue, to which several of my colleagues responded. The chief of pediatrics of a well-known Connecticut hospital wrote:

> I was impressed by your efforts at learning more about chiropractic education as described in the June issue of *Connecticut Medicine*. I echo your concerns about the lack of any scientific evidence demonstrating the effectiveness of chiropractic. As a pediatrician, I am, of course, most concerned about the attempts made to influence parents and care givers as to the need for periodic "adjustments" on children. These have been advertised as being useful in the prevention and treatment of such diverse entities as asthma, enuresis, learning disabilities, and ear infections (to name a few)!
>
> Following the appearance of several "glitzy" ads by local chiropractors claiming positive results in these areas, I wrote and contacted our state's Office of Health and Consumer Affairs. This was felt by me to be a clear example of false advertising and the individuals who were responsible for these ads have stopped (temporarily?) publishing them. However, no further investi-

gation or attempts on limiting these practices were pursued.

I would be most interested to see if your efforts have reaped any benefits. I agree that the cost of such unproven treatments are astronomical and that the medical profession is bearing an undue burden by having most of these treatments and manipulations covered through various health insurance plans. This is an issue that should not be left unexamined.

Another medical colleague, just as serious, but in a different vein sent me an essay written by the late H.L. Mencken, which is reprinted in Chapter 4.

The president of New York Chiropractic College, Kenneth W. Padgett, DC, responded:

Concerning the legitimacy of chiropractic, I believe it is important to call your readers' attention to the fact that there have been internationally recognized studies regarding the efficacy of chiropractic care. The first was an in-depth study conducted in the early 1990s by the Rand Corporation. This study revealed that spinal manipulation is of benefit to patients with acute low back pain. It is interesting to note that this study was conducted by a team of medical doctors as well as doctors of chiropractic. The second study, concluded in 1994, was a publication of patient guidelines by the U.S. Department of Health and Human Services Agency for Health Care Policy Research (AHCPR). This document recommended manipulation as the preferred therapy for low back pain in adults.

At New York Chiropractic College, we provide our students a quality education. This is readily evidenced by the fact that the college holds an Absolute Charter from the New York State Board of Regents and is accredited by the Commission on Accreditation of the Council on Chiropractic Education to award the Doctor of Chiropractic degree. New York Chiropractic College is also regionally accredited by the Commission on Higher Education, Middle States Association of Colleges and Schools.

We are proud of the high level of achievement our graduates attain as health care providers. Our students are well-trained in diagnosis and, as practitioners, know what to treat within their scope of practice and know when to refer to other health care professionals. The renewed health of literally tens of thousands of satisfied patients provides living testimony to the effectiveness of chiropractic care.

In closing, I would like to affirm the college's commitment to seeking the best health care possible for those persons we are committed to serve. We believe it is imperative for all health care providers to work together, and we would welcome visits to our campus from those who are interested in joining this vital undertaking.

I was given the courtesy of replying to this letter, as is a common practice of medical journals. Among other things, I pointed out that President Padgett could not answer the basic questions that I posed in my visit to the college. Namely, just what is chiropractic supposed to be, and just what is the chiropractic theory? He did not, nor did anyone at the college, give any proof for the existence of a "subluxation" of a spinal vertebra pressing on a nerve, interfering with the passage of energy down that nerve and causing disease to organs supplied by that nerve. To this basic question, I replied, the evidence is that chiropractic does not, by such definition, exist.

I also commented on the AHCPR findings so proudly touted by chiropractic and President Padgett and pointed out that, first of all, the study did not even mention the word chiropractic but simply spoke of spinal manipulation, which osteopaths, physiotherapists, as well as chiropractors practice. I pointed out that the whole findings were based primarily on a meta-analysis done by Dr. Paul Schekelle of California, who had been engaged by the Rand Corporation, which was paid $1 million by the California Chiropractic Association to study this problem.

The study did show a small percentage of decrease in the recovery time in those whose spines were manipulated for low back pain, but this only applied to manipulations between the second and fourth weeks of acute low back pain and was ineffective before 2 weeks and ineffective after 4 weeks. I also should have pointed out that the guidelines show that manipulation is probably harmful when sciatica is caused by a ruptured intervertebral disk. In such cases, manipulation can cause cauda equina syndrome, a condition in which damage to the nerves near the lower end of the spine causes weakness of the legs and loss of bladder and bowel control.

I further pointed out that a more recent study by a Finnish group suggested that having patients twist their spines laterally to each side and backwards and forwards 10 times each every hour throughout the day until their back recovered made recovery longer than for those who simply walked about and did nothing beyond tolerance, which tends to negate the AHCPR findings. Finally, I reminded the readers that most back pains recover spontaneously at the end of 4 weeks regardless of treatment and that some 80% of ruptured disks did so also without surgery. The Rand report and AHCPR guidelines are discussed in more detail in Chapter 18.

Although the precise cause and the best treatment for low back pain are unclear, one dictum that seems to be gaining credence is "leave the back alone and it will get better on its own"—in most cases. If this is true, then chiropractic now has no claims for valid scientific evidence for treating anything. Certainly it does not take 5 or 6 years of some sort of college education to manipulate the spine, for which individual chiropractors apparently develop their own techniques. There is no specific knowledge of exactly what is being manipulated, what it is supposed to do, and specific guidelines as to how to do it, based on science.

Chiropractor Padgett wrote in his letter to the editor, "Our students are well trained in diagnosis." It is incomprehensible how he could make such a claim when chiropractic students experience no training inside a hospital where sick people are diagnosed and treated for a wide variety of specific diseases. Medical students, on the other hand, spend 2 or more years of hospital clinical ward work diagnosing and dealing with the sick, whereas most chiropractic students concentrate on learning how to diagnose and treat "subluxations." Furthermore, most medical school graduates complete at least 3 more years of hospital-based postgraduate training—followed by a lifetime of continuing medical education.

Also, many chiropractors who claim all or most disease is caused by spinal misalignments feel little need to search for a specific diagnosis. Their primary or exclusive treatment is a chiropractic "adjustment" of the spine.

Based on this claim that they are diagnosticians, chiropractors have lobbied to be considered primary care physicians under managed care programs. They claim to be able to diagnose and treat some diseases and to refer the others to medical doctors. Based on the limited training experience in chiropractic college, it would appear that they are qualified to do neither.

If President Padgett wishes to achieve the goal stated in his letter to the editor that he "would like to confirm the college's commitment to seeking the best health care possible for those persons we are committed to serve," he would be well advised to consider the conversion of New York Chiropractic College into an accredited medical school as I suggested to the dean when I visited his college.

The following is my letter to the editor in response to Dr. Padgett:

> The letter by chiropractor Kenneth W. Padgett, president of New York Chiropractic College, fails to address the very basic questions posed during my visit to the college, namely, where is the evidence for the chiropractic theory that there is a "subluxation" of a spine

vertebra which presses on a nerve, interfering with the passage of energy down that nerve to an organ and causing disease of that organ, and further, where is the evidence that chiropractic "adjustments" can benefit or cure these diseases? In scientific terms, what are the names of the diseases; exactly what is an "adjustment" manipulation and its function? This is the challenge to chiropractic.

As for the RAND report and the controversial Agency for the Health Care Policy and Research guideline report, they were both based primarily on the meta-analysis of Paul G. Shekelle et al, funded by the California Chiropractic Foundation. The AHCPR panel consisting of two osteopaths, two chiropractors, 11 medical doctors, and eight others, found that spinal manipulation was not helpful in the first two weeks of acute low-back pain, or after four weeks for chronic pain. There was a statistical increase in the rate of recovery associated with manipulation only in the two-week window period between the second and fourth week, at the end of which time back pain disappeared in most cases regardless of the treatment given.

Neither does the Padgett letter mention the RAND finding that, "serious complications of lumbar manipulation, including paraplegia and death, have been reported."

Manipulations were performed by osteopaths, medical doctors, and chiropractors, but nowhere in the whole AHCPR report does the word chiropractic appear.

A subsequent report which tends to negate these findings, which president Padgett failed to address, is the Helsinki report of 9 February 1995 appearing in the *New England Journal of Medicine*. A group of low-back patients were instructed to twist their backs from one side to the other and backwards, 10 times each, every hour to their limit of pain tolerance. The group subjected to these spine-stretching exercises took longer to recover than a control group who had nothing done to their backs and simply went about their usual activities of daily living to tolerance.

More importantly and to the point, the theory of chiropractic and its claims to be a legitimate method of providing a variety of health care far exceeds the boundaries of controversial spinal manipulation limited to the third or fourth week of low-back pain. For example, chiropractic claims to be able to effectively treat ear infections with cervical manipulative adjustments, and that every newborn must have prompt and periodic spinal adjustments. This must be challenged as wishful thinking or pure quackery. And so, my impression of a visit to a chiropractic college remains the same. Clearly, there is no evidence for such an entity as chiropractic as defined, and their colleges should abandon the outmoded theory and be converted into scientific medical schools.

Another letter to the editor came from Timothy C. Merrick, Board of Directors, Connecticut Chiropractic Council:

I read with a mixture of mirth and sadness the letter by Mr. Chotkowski in the June issue of *Connecticut Medicine* regarding his review of Chiropractic in general and New York Chiropractic College specifically. My mirth was elicited by Mr. Chotkowski's unbridled bias against, and appalling ignorance of, the science, art and philosophy of chiropractic. While it is not uncommon to witness this kind of hard-line, dogmatic attitude — regardless of the reams of research published in the last 20 years — there are few who will unabashedly parade their prejudice like Mr. Chotkowski.

My sadness came from the fact that *Connecticut Medicine*—an otherwise worthy publication—would print a letter like his. Mr. Chotkowski's glaring lack of objectivity flies in the face of responsible journalism.

For instance: Mr. Chotkowski suggests that New York Chiropractic College had no research department. Obviously, he did not care to ask. He also did not care to find out that indeed the library was well equipped with scientific journals. He suggests that the chiropractic curriculum is a three year program when it is a ten semester program with over 4900 credit hours of didactic and practical education — on par with medical college programs. While he took the time to go to the college, he did not apparently take the time to learn anything. I believe his *modus operandi* was, "don't confuse me with the truth."

The biggest problem that Mr. Chotkowski seemed to have was understanding that chiropractic works from a different paradigm than medicine. To compare chiropractic with medicine is like apples and oranges. He was right, we do not "diagnose and treat specific diseases." That is the practice of medicine. Is his world so small that nothing can exist outside of this realm?

Chiropractic focuses on the connection between structure and function. Specifically between the spine and the function of the nervous system. The aim of chiropractic is not to treat disease but to detect and correct vertebral subluxation; to remove that which interferes with the innate healing capacity of the human body. As it happens, numerous studies show the beneficial effects of this type of care on people who suffer from many different disease conditions. Suggesting that there is no evidence to support the "theory" of chiropractic leads one to believe that it is Mr. Chotkowski's library that is devoid of scientific journals.

Mr. Chotkowski would like to see the elimination of the chiropractic profession. Need we remind him of the United States Supreme Court ruling against the American Medical Association for trying to do just that?

Since that landmark decision to uphold a lower court's guilty verdict against the AMA, there has been an ever-increasing, constructive dialogue between medical doctors and chiropractors. I personally work with several physicians who refer patients to this office for chiropractic care. Patients who suffer from conditions ranging from low back pain to otitis media. They refer *because they have found that their patients benefit from the referral.* This bridge between our professions only serves to help our patients. Mr. Chotkowski's false and inflammatory letter—and your printing of it—is damaging to this bridge and does not serve any productive purpose.

I hope to see more constructive and objective articles in future issues.

Respectfully,
Dr. Timothy C. Merrick, DC

I responded:

Dear Editor:
Chiropractor Timothy Merrick's letter apparently expresses the view of the Connecticut Chiropractic Council, and again reveals the true nature of the chiropractic dilemma. The letter states that chiropractic admittedly "cannot diagnose and treat specific disease," and that the "aim is not to treat disease but to detect and correct vertebral subluxations." The problem with that aim is that the existence of a subluxation has never been demonstrated and all scientific evidence of its existence is to the contrary. In fact, the recent attempt of the 16 college presidents even to define a subluxation falls short of any clear description of it, as follows:

"Subluxation is a complex of functional and/or structural and/or pathological changes that compromise neural integrity and may influence organ system's function and health. A subluxation is evaluated, diagnosed and managed through use of chiropractic procedures based on the best available rational empirical evidence"—terms that have been described as "chiroprattle."

As for *Wilk vs. AMA* [the Supreme Court case to which Merrick had referred], Federal Judge Susan Getzendanner did not find chiropractic to be a valid health care system but only that it was illegal for the AMA to engage in an antitrust boycott of a licensed practice.

Regarding the creation of a constructive dialogue and bridging the gap between unscientific chiropractic and scientific medicine, the quickest way this can be accomplished is for chiropractic to abandon its ludicrous theory and convert its colleges into accredited medical schools—as osteopaths have done.

A third letter was received from chiropractor Luigi DiRubba as follows:

I found it outrageous that you chose to print the letter from L.A. Chotkowski, M.D. in your June 1997 (Letter to the Editor) column.

By saying he was already convinced that chiropractic was a "medical hoax," he admitted that he was visiting New York Chiropractic College with a completely closed mind and intentional antagonism.

What purpose does it serve to air the "opinions" of a man who not only is closed minded, but seems to revel in his intolerance? Wouldn't your readers and your profession be better served by exposure to opinions from those within your ranks who approach the topic of non-medical health care from an unbiased opinion and possible self interest?

There are thousands of medical doctors around the country and the world who are opening their minds to the countless possibilities offered by nonmedical approaches to "health care", including nutrition, acupuncture and yes, Chiropractic.

These are true health professionals who are not driven by fear or hatred; but who have recognized the limits of their own understanding and want to learn as well as promote and teach. They are overcoming decades of AMA initiated antichiropractic propaganda and are now working very closely with chiropractors to provide a full range of health care services to their patients.

They are also coming to understand—as Dr. Chotkowski apparently does not — that chiropractic is not a "medical hoax" or even a "medical" treatment. In fact, it does not offer treatments, symptom relief, or cures. Its sole purpose is the totally nonmedical one of correcting vertebral subluxations (yes, Doc, there is such a thing—just review the scientific literature within the past 20 years) to allow the human body to function better. It has been called the most conservative and, therefore, the safest of *all* health care approaches. Why does Dr. Chotkowski—or any medical doctor feel threatened by this? What does he or she have to lose, other than patients who leave his/her office with nothing more than a prescription?

Chiropractic has not grown to become the second largest health-care field in the world based on a giant "HOAX." It has grown and will continue to grow, because patients want one alternative to the often frustrating failure of "medical treatments" to safely and effectively help them achieve health and wellness.

If Dr. Chotkowski resents or fears its growth, then he should look at the weaknesses inherent in his own profession rather than trying to discredit or destroy the "competition."

Dr. Chotkowski also says he introduced a bill which would have banned the use of chiropractic on children and any manipulation of the neck, presumably because in his opinion (that has no factual basis) these practices pose some sort of "danger" to the public. Might I suggest that he research the literature on this issue and also read the medical literature on iatrogenic diseases and deaths which claim the health and lives of hundreds of thousands of people each year. What law will he introduce to put a stop to the tragedy?

Your publication has a responsibility to its readers and to the public they serve. Do not relinquish that responsibility by printing hate-mongering diatribes which clearly do not adhere to even the lowest standards of professional objectivity or journalistic ethics.

Luigi DiRubba, D.C. (Chiropractor)

My response:

Chiropractor Luigi DiRubba's letter reveals the dilemma in which chiropractic finds itself today, namely there is no scientific evidence for the chiropractic theory of "subluxation" of a spinal vertebra pressing on a nerve that can be adjusted to treat or prevent disease.

In what appears to be an admission of this, the letter states, "In fact, it (chiropractic) does not offer treatments, symptom relief, or cures." What apparently remains of chiropractic then is the claim that a theoretical adjustment of a vertebra can "achieve wellness." If this is not a "giant hoax," then at least it is a giant medical oxymoron.

As for DiRubba's claim that chiropractic manipulation of the cervical spine is without danger, the 1994 *Consumer Reports* states that a prominent malpractice insurance company paid some 140 claims for chiropractic-induced strokes in one year. This alone should call for legislative consideration of a bill to ban licensure at least for cervical manipulation of adults, and a bill will be introduced again this year.

One issue avoided in his letter is the cost of chiropractic care. Based on 70,000 chiropractors in the U.S. today, the cost of chiropractors' and chiropractic assistants' incomes, office, radiology, and laboratory expenses of some 200 to 300 thousand dollars each, the total cost is about 14 to 21 billion dollars a year—a massive health-care cost for a scientifically unproven entity.

The chairman of the Connecticut Sports Medicine Committee wrote in a very supportive letter, "I compliment you on exposing yourself to the bombastics of the chiropractic community. You are right. There is a massive health care cost for an unproven entity but certainly a widely publicized entity." He expressed concern that insurance companies were paying for referrals to the neurological chiropractor, the sports medicine chiropractor, and the exercise physiologist chiropractor. He expressed concern in the following statement: "I am not sure where this will ever end up but again I compliment you on your efforts."

The Clinic at Bridgeport

To gain broader knowledge about what is being taught in chiropractic colleges, I visited the University of Bridgeport College of Chiropractic in Bridgeport, Connecticut. The college is 10 years old and has about 250 students. The admission requirements are 3 years of prechiropractic preparation. The total tuition and expense cost is about $13,000 per year for 4 years. It is the only university-affiliated chiropractic college in the United States.

A student guide was assigned to me for a tour of the buildings, which appeared adequate. I particularly wished to visit the college's clinic and view firsthand the performance of a spinal "adjustment" of a "vertebral subluxation." No patient was available, so the clinic director approved of my guide volunteering as a patient.

My guide then lay face-down on a low table with his face cradled in a hole in one end to allow breathing. The student adjuster then felt each side of the patient's neck and reported finding a cervical "subluxation" under his fingers. He then examined the thoracic and lumber spines in the same manner, finding a "subluxation" in each.

Grasping the patient's head with both hands, he hyper-extended his head, twisted it to one side, and suddenly gave a series of jerks. He then repeated the twists and jerks on the other side, completing the cervical "adjustment." The procedure struck me as a form of hanging without a rope or gallows. I could only wonder what damage such twisting might be doing to the carotid and vertebral arteries serving the brain, as well as damage to the intervetebral disks.

The adjuster then turned the patient on his side, flexed the higher leg, clasped the leg and the thorax region, and gave a series of vigorous thrusts. The patient was then turned over and the thrusts repeated.

When the "adjustments" were completed, the adjuster asked whether I had heard the cracks and assured me that they were only the sound of gas escaping from the joints.

Following this shocking demonstration of a chiropractic "adjustment," I visited the dean and asked him to name the exact diseases that students were taught this procedure could effectively treat. His answer was similar to the "wellness" answer given by the dean of New York Chiropractic College. Students were being taught to how treat the "patient."

When I challenged this "patient" concept, he suggested that I read the writings of Anthony Rosner, PhD, a spokesman for chiropractic. I responded that if he would turn on the computer on his desk, he could find on Rosner's Web site my scientific medical reply to Rosner's essay on the treatment of otitis media.

He then brought out a book written by Walter I. Wardwell for me to read. I responded that Wardwell, a professor of sociology at the University of Connecticut, had just written his last piece of advice to the chiropractic community, recommending that they get their act together and that different factions and beliefs unite into a single definition and practice of chiropractic.

The dean quietly put the book aside and handed me a copy of the latest chiropractic paradigm described in Chapter 1 of this book. After a few cordial exchanges, the visit ended.

11
Visit with an
Alaskan Chiropractor

In August 1997, I went on a fly-fishing trip in Alaskan bush country with my son and two grandsons. Our base connection to civilization was Dillingham, Alaska, a center for the salmon fishing industry in Bristol Bay.

Right in the middle of this small, quiet, rustic fishing village was a sign declaring the Chiropractic Family Health Center. Following a wonderful trip of catching loads of giant rainbows, dolly varden, king, silver, and sockeye salmon—all release fishing—we returned to Dillingham before flying home. I noticed the chiropractic center was open and decided to visit.

The chiropractor was busy with a patient as I sat in the small waiting room. I noted chiropractic pamphlets in the office and the standard chiropractic spinal chart depicting vertebrae and spinal nerves going to various organs. When the chiropractor finally appeared, I stated that I was here from Connecticut on a fishing trip, was writing a book about chiropractic, and was interested in what he was doing way up in Alaskan bush country. I also mentioned the proposed name of the book, citing its provocative title.

The chiropractor was an affable, friendly man in his early 30s by appearance and quite willing to be interviewed for my book. He said that the major problems in his area, populated largely by native Alaskans, were alcoholism and boredom. I was unable to get a clear picture of exactly what health problems he was treating, but he did say there was a small hospital in the area where he referred patients from time to time if he felt they were too sick for him to manage. There was also a free immunization clinic for children in the town. I asked about his position on immunization. He said he did not advise patients against immunization, but he, himself, was opposed and did not immunize his own children—a position midway in the chiropractic spectrum of attitudes toward immunization.

I questioned why he had chosen chiropractic over a medical career. He replied that his college grades had not been good enough to get into medical school and that his applications to dental schools had been rejected.

After pointing out that, in my view, chiropractic could not treat any disease, I asked whether he would not feel better giving scientific medical care to his patients instead of chiropractic. He replied that he was happy keeping them healthy with "adjustments."

I then asked whether he would consider returning to medical school if his college and other chiropractic colleges would convert to such medical schools. He replied that medical school of 2 years and especially 2 more years of internship would be too long. He was quite interested in this concept, however, and mentioned that Western States Chiropractic College, in Portland, Oregon, was considering such a change.

We debated the issue of unscientific chiropractic, and he pointed out a pamphlet about the Agency for Health Care Policy and Research (AHCPR) report, prominently displayed in his waiting room. I replied that the report was an outcome meta-analysis (these are subject to error) and that the guidelines mentioned only manipulation and stretching back structures but did not validate chiropractic subluxation theory. I also mentioned the recent Finnish randomized outcome study that largely negated the Shekelle meta-analysis on which the AHCPR guidelines were largely based.

He had the last word in this debate, assuring me that he was happy with his work among the Alaskan bush country people and was providing them with good chiropractic care.

Following the visit, I had time to review the various pamphlets I obtained in his office. Of particular interest were those issued by the Parker Chiropractic Research Foundation

(PCRF) on kidney trouble, liver trouble, subluxation, headache, ulcers, whiplash, high blood pressure, and childhood ear infections. These appear to be the same type of pamphlets issued some 30 years ago by the same organization mentioned in Ralph Smith's book on chiropractic.

To a medical-science oriented person like myself, these pamphlets all seem to be masterpieces of obfuscation. For example, the pamphlet entitled "Kidney Trouble" does not use "diseases" because it does not dicuss any specific kidney disease, such as glomerulonephritis, polycystic kidney disease, or even kidney stones. Rather, the pamphlet states:

> The body has two kidneys. They lie at the lower border
> of the rib cage, on each side of the spinal column. The
> waste material from the kidney is drained into a central
> location—the bladder—to be eliminated.

All very true, so far. However, the section on "Symptoms of Kidney Trouble" states incorrectly that the most commonly recognized symptom is an aching sensation in the small of the back. Most kidney disease is either painless or, in the case of obstruction or stones, causes pain in either costovertebral angle or the abdomen. Now comes the chiropractic pitch in the pamphlet, which is, in my view, quite false: "The most common cause of kidney trouble is inadequate function due to improper nerve supply." The truth is that kidney function is controlled by hormonal mechanisms, and an adequate blood supply and has nothing to do with its nerve supply. Kidneys can function perfectly well with no nerve supply at all—as demonstrated by transplanted kidneys, which are separated from their nerve supply when removed from the donor's body.

The obfuscation continues with the claim that the nervous system is a master system of the body and controls the function of other systems, including elimination. The pamphlet then describes the brain and spinal cord and claims that misaligned vertebrae interfere with normal function of the nervous system and "can thereby stress the immune system, putting the body in a weakened state that can set the stage for all kinds of malfunction—kidney trouble included." These are all chiropractic assumptions and unproven claims in the view of medical science. The next section of the "Kidney Trouble" pamphlet, titled "Treatment," states:

> The standard medical approach to kidney problems varies depending upon the severity of the condition. In mild to moderate cases, diuretic drugs, antibiotics and other medication are usually prescribed to increase function and combat infection. If the condition fails to improve or worsens, various other procedures are used, including mechanical dialysis. Finally, if the problem still doesn't improve or worsens, surgery is often resorted to including a kidney transplant.
>
> Chiropractic is neither a kidney therapy nor a treatment for kidney trouble, yet patients with kidney problems are turning to their neighborhood chiropractors in record numbers and chiropractors have a high level of patient satisfaction.

The final two paragraphs, which appear almost verbatim in just about all the pamphlets, read as follows:

> Chiropractors are health care professionals highly trained to analyze the spinal column for vertebral subluxations that cause nerve irritation—the most common underlying cause of kidney trouble. Today the vertebral subluxation has reached epidemic proportions. This condition is called a "silent killer" because at the same time it is weakening the body and paving the way for diseases, people may be entirely unaware they have a problem.
>
> If vertebral subluxations are found, the chiropractor uses special techniques (without drugs or surgery) to correct the subluxation and relieve the nerve irritation. This is called a chiropractic adjustment. The purpose of the chiropractic spinal adjustment is to remove

nerve irritation, thus permitting the body to restore itself to a greater level of energy and health.

The "Liver Trouble" pamphlet and other pamphlets are written in the same manner, some truth mixed with unproven theory and unproven statements, all suggesting that chiropractors can prevent or treat diseases of organs while correctly denying, at the same time, that chiropractic can treat any specific organ disease. It would seem that one reason such pamphlets must be carefully written so as not to be false advertising is the danger of using the mail to defraud, and chiropractic must stay within the boundaries of its unproven theory.

The claim in that patients are satisfied with chiropractic treatment—whatever that is—is correct to a degree, although there are many who are dissatisfied. Frankly, it is difficult to understand why anyone would want to be treated with spinal manipulation for a serious disease.

The Dillingham chiropractor was very interested in my book and wanted to know whether he would be in it. He seemed pleased that I said yes and appeared to feel that he had handled the problem of chiropractic adroitly. Perhaps to have the last word and ensure that his viewpoint was registered, he wrote the following letter a few weeks later addressed to me as L.A. Chotkowski, RD (real doctor):

> Dear Sir:
> Thank you for reaffirming my belief in the chiropractic subluxation. Having jerks like you re-ignites my duty to let people know that allopathic medicine is run by the pharmaceutical giants. You guys treat symptoms, not the cause of disease. Maybe you should go back to chiropractic college and learn a thing or two.
> Sincerely.

It seems that chiropractic theory and philosophy are alive and well ingrained throughout the nation, including Alaskan bush country.

12

A Chiropractic Lecture
on Headache

On a rainy summer evening, I and a medical colleague attended a public lecture given at a West Hartford, Connecticut, library by a local chiropractor on the subject of headaches. We signed in and joined some 12 enthusiastic attendees, most of whom professed, by a show of hands when asked by the lecturer, to have suffered a headache at some time or other. I also raised my hand on this issue.

The lecture, I soon discerned, was based on the practice-building strategies mentioned in previous chapters of this book.

The speaker, in a very congenial and pleasant manner, began by explaining how we all have headaches periodically. He then proceeded to describe the types of headache in a fairly accurate manner, covering the subject as found in any medical textbook and based on scientific knowledge. However, he also brought out the typical chiropractic spinal column model, displayed in many chiropractic offices and advertisements, and proceeded to point out the area where "subluxations" were pressing on nerves, causing symptoms of headache.

He then described how spinal "adjustments" relieved these symptoms. In doing so, he criticized the medical profession for only "treating symptoms" with Advil, Tylenol, or aspirin, whereas chiropractors, by relieving the pressure on the nervous system, "treat the cause." It is like prescribing an antacid for indigestion, he explained, which treats the symptoms, whereas spinal "adjustments" get at the cause. He did not explain exactly how this was accomplished physiologically, except to say that the nervous system in the spine controlled all body functions and that his manipulations were a natural way of treating the disease.

He showed a series of anatomical drawings of the spine, projected on a screen, to explain the chiropractic theory that pinching of spinal nerves produced headaches. Then—out of the blue—he showed a diagram of a child passing through the birth canal, which he described as "very tight," and said that twisting and pulling of the child's neck during delivery produced cervical "subluxations." These had to be adjusted, he warned, or else the child might suffer sudden infant death syndrome. He also claimed that the child would need treatments immediately and all throughout life to stay healthy. Nobody in the audience took exception to these imaginative statements.

The chiropractor then produced a "Chiropractic Research Chart" (see page 107) from among several pieces of chiropractic literature in a packet given to each participant. A similar chart from the Parker Chiropractic Research Foundation was mentioned in *At Your Own Risk* in 1969.

Such charts are interesting because they suggest that chiropractic treatment can help people with an enormous range of symptoms and conditions. These charts do not state when or how the figures were compiled, how the diagnoses were made, what treatment was given, how many patients were allegedly studied, or how the patient evaluations were obtained. Many of the categories are not specific conditions but are symptoms or groups of conditions. Some of the figures are preposterous. If spinal adjustments could cure or substantially improve 81.9% of patients with kidney disease, 80.5% of patients with liver disorders, or 80.9% of those with gallbladder disease, they would be making headlines everywhere—and perhaps Andy Warhol would still be alive today. No medical journal would publish such an undocumented and irresponsible report, but nobody in the audience appeared to find anything wrong with it.

Following his formal presentation, the chiropractor held what he termed a "workshop," in which the audience participated. He asked everyone to stand; raise their arms; inhale

CHIROPRACTIC RESEARCH CHART

These statistics represent the results obtained under chiropractic care for a large variety of chronic conditions. The vast majority of these cases had also been previously diagnosed and treated by practitioners other than Doctors of Chiropractic.

Condition	Accepted* for Treatment	Well or Much Improved	Slightly Improved	Same	Continued to Worsen
Allergies	92.3%	87.2%	10.3%	2.5%	0%
Arm & Leg Pain	92.1%	88.2%	5.2%	6.0%	.6%
Arthritis	89.2%	73.3%	16.8%	9.4%	.5%
Asthma	92.3%	80.5%	12.1%	6.5%	.9%
Bronchitis	94.3%	84.2%	9.9%	3.9%	2.0%
Bursitis	96.1%	89.3%	7.1%	3.6%	0%
Chest Pains	93.2%	91.0%	7.1%	1.9%	0%
Constipation	98.3%	79.2%	13.3%	6.7%	.8%
Dizziness	94.6%	86.3%	7.8%	5.9%	0%
Gallbladder Disorders	90.3%	80.9%	11.3%	5.8%	2.0%
General Tension	86.4%	72.5%	16.5%	8.8%	2.2%
General Weakness	89.2%	87.0%	8.7%	0%	4.3%
Hay fever	92.3%	81.6%	13.4%	5.0%	0%
Headache, non-migraine	98.7%	83.2%	11.1%	5.1%	.6%
Herniated Discs	87.3%	88.2%	7.9%	3.5%	.4%
High Blood Pressure	88.6%	73.0%	19.3%	6.4%	1.3%
Indigestion	96.4%	89.4%	4.5%	5.3%	.8%
Insomnia	94.6%	81.8%	11.4%	5.1%	1.7%
Joint Pain	96.1%	82.2%	9.7%	8.1%	0%
Kidney Disorders	88.3%	81.9%	3.6%	9.7%	4.8%
Liver Disorders	87.1%	80.5%	11.7%	5.8%	2.0%
Low Back Problems	96.7%	87.3%	8.0%	4.2%	.5%
Low Blood Pressure	94.1%	73.6%	17.6%	7.8%	1.0%
Menopause Disorders	87.1%	73.4%	13.3%	11.3%	2.0%
Menstrual Disorders	94.6%	81.8%	11.9%	5.9%	4.0%
Migraine Headaches	93.6%	86.6%	8.1%	2.9%	2.4%
Nausea	84.2%	87.2%	10.3%	2.5%	0%
Nervousness	95.6%	80.8%	12.8%	5.3%	1.1%
Neuralgia	97.3%	80.1%	14.2%	5.7%	0%
Neuritis	98.2%	86.4%	6.4%	7.2%	0%
Numbness in Hands or Feet	90.4%	85.5%	8.0%	5.5%	1.0%
Rheumatism	96.1%	77.2%	14.7%	8.1%	0%
Sacroiliac Disorders	98.4%	81.8%	17.2%	1.0%	0%
Sciatica	97.2%	85.0%	9.4%	5.1%	.5%
Sinusitis	93.1%	83.2%	11.8%	4.7%	.3%
Slipped Disc	94.2%	88.7%	7.9%	3.0%	.4%
Spinal Curvatures	97.1%	82.9%	5.7%	8.6%	2.8%
Stiff Necks	92.6%	93.2%	4.4%	2.4%	0%
Stomach Disorders	91.3%	82.5%	13.1%	3.7%	.7%

Doctors of chiropractic do not accept all cases but help nearly all they accept.

deeply; close their eyes; exhale and relax; and then turn their head this way, then that way, forward, and backward. Then he asked, "Now don't you all feel better," to which everyone but my colleague and I responded, "Yes."

I gathered that the purpose of this exercise was to subtly suggest that neck manipulation was safe and beneficial. Then the chiropractor had the group act alternately as doctor and patient by massaging and gently tilting each other's heads to break down any barriers of fear and to further promote the chiropractic concept.

When the audience participation was over, he offered a free consultation and examination to "anyone signing up tonight but not thereafter." He then opened the meeting to questions and answers. After one person asked a question and there appeared to be no more, I asked whether he had actually ever seen a subluxation. He seemed taken aback by this question but claimed that the wonderful results of chiropractic proved that subluxations existed.

"But," I persisted, "have you ever seen one by autopsy, surgery, x-ray, CT scan or other imaging technique?"

"By x-ray," was his answer.

"But x-rays don't show subluxations or nerves. Even Scott Haldeman calls it a functional spinal lesion, not an anatomical one, in his book."

The audience became a bit restless at this point and began to speak up in his defense, voicing objections to my questioning and saying that chiropractic helped them. I persisted with one more question, "You said much about the dangers of medicine and surgery, but what about the dangers of chiropractic neck manipulation? Do you inform your patients that neck adjustments can cause strokes and even be fatal?"

"It doesn't happen," he replied.

"Well," I said, "you must certainly have heard about chiropractor Thomas Goulding of Waterford, who was judged responsible for causing the stroke of Linda Solsbury, who now lies completely paralyzed in a hospital here in New Britain.

Goulding was successfully sued for $10 million." At this point, the audience protested further and the meeting ended.

Two audience members came up to me later, and one said, "I've been going to a chiropractor for neck adjustments for 20 years and nothing has ever happened to me."

"What's your problem?" I asked.

"I was injured and had a ruptured disk in my neck."

"How come you still have the problem after 20 years of chiropractic and didn't have an operation that could have cured your disk overnight?" I asked.

"I'm afraid of surgery," he replied.

The other member asked whether I was a doctor and said, "I have headaches every month and have been going to my regular doctor and still have them, and I would like a cure."

I hesitated to get involved in this manner, but I was curious about her story and why she had come to the lecture.

"Do they come with your periods?" I asked. "Yes," she said, and went on to describe the classical symptoms of migraine.

"Well," I said, "there are a number of medications your doctor may have tried like diuretics for premenstrual tension syndrome and fluid retention, Inderal, or the newer serotonin inhibitor, sumatriptan, sold as Imitrex."

"Oh yes," she said, "he prescribed Imitrex but if I don't take it right away, it doesn't work. I still suffer sometimes every month and I would like a cure."

In leaving the meeting, I said to the chiropractor who was attending the refreshments, "Nothing personal, you understand, just wanted to ask a few questions."

I left with my medical colleague, who had informed me of the meeting. He commented, as we were walking out, "These people all seem as though they are hypnotized. Once they are programmed to believe something, no amount of reasoning or fact can dissuade them or convince them otherwise."

So true, I agreed, and so ended the lesson.

13
Additional Opinions
about Chiropractic

While preparing the first edition of this book, I sent the following letter to a leading chiropractic organization and several well-known experts.

> Dear Member of the Scientific Community,
> I am writing a book titled *Chiropractic, the Greatest Hoax of the Century?*, which concludes that, "there is no such entity as the chiropractic theory of subluxation of a spinal vertebra, pressing on a nerve, causing disease of various organs supplied by that nerve, and that concludes that chiropractic adjustments of such theoretical subluxations cannot alleviate disease or maintain health." I am seeking opinions from various prominent authorities and organizations in the scientific field that would support this view, and would appreciate an opinion from you.

The first response came from Anthony L. Rosner, PhD, (biochemistry), director of research for the Foundation for Chiropractic Education and Research, a group that funds chiropractic studies but also issues a considerable amount of propaganda:

> Dear Dr. Chotkowski:
> I am in receipt of your letter of August 26th seeking an opinion in support of your view that chiropractic may be the greatest hoax of the century. As the Director of Research for a foundation with over a 50-year history for supporting peer-reviewed research pertaining to chiropractic, I find your viewpoint disappointing in its

failure to grasp not only several goals and accomplishments of chiropractic research, but also how *medical* procedures are often practiced without scientific documentation.

I can appreciate your impatience with attempts to define the term "subluxation"; indeed, there are varying opinions both within and outside the chiropractic community as to precisely what the term denotes. For your reference, I have enclosed a copy of a recent monograph that I have devoted to just that subject — and you will note that there has been a gradual evolution of a suitable definition of the term with only a recent consensus within the chiropractic community, and numerous research efforts have established with varying degrees of success our working concepts of the term. For you to condemn the term outright, however, seems as futile and ill-advised as if you were to condemn quantum mechanics simply because it attempts to advance our understanding of matter by describing its wavelike properties in addition to its more commonly accepted particulate nature.

Your describing chiropractic as a hoax flies in the face of leading government reports from both the United States [1] and Great Britain [2], which unequivocally state that chiropractic is one of the *leading* alternatives in the management of back pain *and* that these conclusions are based upon the fact that the evidence for the effectiveness of chiropractic is among the strongest of any of the health professions reviewed. This recognition could not have been possible under the terms of your current assessment of chiropractic.

First, one must be aware that only 15% of *medical* procedures have been documented in any way in the peer-reviewed scientific literature [3], only 1% of which has been deemed to be methodologically sound [4]. Coronary bypass surgery, glaucoma surgery, and many procedures in orthopedic surgery were initiated with virtually no literature to support them; you would do well to recall that *mainstream* medicine, held before us as the gold standard, has occasionally endorsed such ill-advised and short-lived therapies as the use of leeches or laughing gas.

Finally, physicians need to be aware that a considerable body of empirical evidence in support of the chiropractic management of such varied conditions as dysmenorrhea [5], premenstrual syndrome [6], otitis media [7], colic [8], enuresis [9], hypertension [10], and asthma [11] does exist in the peer-reviewed literature. Fifteen to twenty years ago, one could say that relatively little refereed literature existed in support of the chiropractic management of back pain. With the passage of time and considerable research, we now know that the medical community, with your unfortunate exception, is beginning to recognize chiropractic management of back pain as a strongly substantiated health care intervention for the treatment of back pain.

Spinal manipulative therapy has been widely regarded as safe and effective for a growing number of conditions in addition to low back pain. Unfortunately, history has shown us that chiropractic has been virulently attacked without basis by many circles in orthodox medicine and the title of your book does give you away as one of the most vociferous exponents of that sentiment that I have ever seen. I hope that you will be able to consider this information that I have sent you before embarking upon what I believe is an ill-informed and ultimately self-defeating undertaking.

References

1. Bigos S, Bowyer O, Braen G, et al. Acute low back pain in adults. Clinical practice guideline No. 14. AHCPR Publication No. 95-0642. Rockville, MD: Agency for Health Care Policy and Research, Public Health Service, U.S. Department of Health and Human Services. December 1994.
2. Rosen M. Back pain. Report of a Clinical Standards Advisory Group Committee on back pain. May 1994, London: HMSO.

3. Smith R. Where is the wisdom? The poverty of medical evidence. British Medical Journal 1991; 303: 798-799.

4. Rachlis N, Kuschner C. Second Opinion: What's Wrong with Canada's Health Care System and How to Fix It, Toronto, ONT: Collins, 1989.

5. Kokjohn K, Schmid DM, Triano JJ, Brennan PC. The effect of spinal manipulation on pain and prostaglandin levels in women with primary dysmenorrhea. Journal of Manipulative and Physiological Therapeutics 1992; 15(5): 279-285.

6. Stude DE. The management of symptoms associated with premenstrual syndrome. Journal of Manipulative and Physiological Therapeutics 1991; 14(3): 209-216.

7. Frohle RM. Ear infection: A retrospective study examining improvement from chiropractic care and analyzing for influencing factors. Journal of Manipulative and Physiological Therapeutics 1996; 19(3):169-177.

8. Klougart N, Nilsson N, Jacobsen J. Infantile colic treated by chiropractors: a prospective study of 316 cases. Journal of Manipulative and Physiological Therapeutics 1989; 12(4): 281-288.

9. Reed WR, Beavers S, Reddy SK, Kern G. Chiropractic management of primary nocturnal enuresis. Journal of Manipulative and Physiological Therapeutics 1994; 17(9):565-600.

10. Yates RG, Lamping DL, Abram NL, Wright C. Effects of chiropractic treatment on blood pressure and anxiety: a randomized, controlled trial. Journal of Manipulative and Physiological Therapeutics 1989; 11(6): 484-488.

11. Hurwitz EL, Aker PD, Adams AH, Meeker WC, Shekelle PG. Manipulation and mobilization of the cervical spine. Spine 1996; 21(15): 1746-1760.

Sincerely yours,

Anthony L. Rosner, PhD

Rosner's letter and enclosed monograph (see excerpts in the following text) display the typical chiropractic dilemma. Chiropractic is unable to clearly define or demonstrate the existence of its "subluxations" or show that its "adjustments" can effectively treat any disease. It therefore must resort to attacks on those engaged in its exposure. For example, in the monograph, *The Role of the Subluxation in Chiropractic*, the most recent attempt to define "subluxation" is as follows:

The term subluxation used by chiropractors to describe altered joint motion, misalignment of articular surfaces and related physiological changes significantly predates the grosser visually cued radiographic subluxation, yet greater than one hundred terms have been proposed to replace the chiropractic subluxation. Changing the name when referring to the manipulable subluxation—whether to manipulable lesion, neurobio-mechanical lesion or orthospondylodysarthritic lesion is no more helpful than calling it a spinal "boo boo," an adjustment seeking lesion, or saying that bad things happen to the spine.

Subluxation has meant an element of misalignment, altered motion, and dysfunction to chiropractors for more than a century. The recent definition of subluxation developed through consensus of the 16 chiropractic college presidents under the auspices of the Association of Chiropractic Colleges in July of 1996 provides a rational and unifying definition for use by the chiropractic profession:

> Subluxation is a complex of functional and/or structural and/or pathologic changes that compromise neural integrity and may influence organ system function and general health. A subluxation is evaluated, diagnosed and managed through the use of chiropractic procedures based on the best available rational and empirical evidence.

It is in this spirit of rationality and unity that I commend this monograph and the use of the term subluxation to both chiropractors and non chiropractors alike.

The monograph Rosner sent me contains contributions from a number of chiropractic college officials offering research studies designed to clarify the meaning of a "subluxation," but nowhere in the text was there a demonstration that it, in fact, exists.

Rosner's letter lists as his No. 1 reference Stanley Bigos, MD, who chaired the Agency for Health Care Policy and Researh (AHCPR) team that developed the guidelines for treating acute low back pain. Curiously, the second response to my inquiry came from Dr. Bigos:

> I received your note of August 26, 1997. I am not totally sure what your note meant exactly, so I will provide you with the recommendations that I have. First of all, as you mentioned, there was no word of chiropractic or the theory of chiropracsy in the AHCPR Guidelines. But due to the fact that there were two articles, one by McDonald and one by Nortin Hadler, that made our evidence tables to show the efficacy above and beyond placebo, it is imperative that we consider manipulation a means of symptom control.
>
> As you might know, symptom control is but one part of care as the real treatment for activity intolerance is conditioning. Speaking strictly for the lumbar spine and not the cervical spine, we had to conclude that lumbar manipulation was safe when there was no significant neurological abnormalities and we had to consider the fact that nobody gets gastrointestinal bleeds from manipulation compared to some of the problems we run into with our nonsteroidal anti-inflammatory medication.
>
> At no point were we able to provide any distinctions related to subluxations causing disease or manipulation correcting a problem. What we could say is that there are a couple of points on a 10-point visual analog scale changed above and beyond placebo with manipulation and that the effect lasted for a few hours. About the same as much less expensive medication methods.
>
> Hope this is helpful.
>
> Sincerely,
> Stanley J. Bigos, MD
> Professor of Orthopedics and
>   Environmental Health
> University of Washington
>   School of Medicine

I interpret Dr. Bigos's reply to mean that the AHCPR panel found no evidence of a "chiropractic subluxation causing disease or manipulation correcting a problem." The text of the guidelines did not even mention chiropractic. The panel evidently considered seriously two studies showing that spinal manipulation gave "a couple of points" of relief of symptoms on a scale of 10 but no cure of the condition.

These two studies showed that the effect of spinal manipulation lasted only for about "a few hours" and was about the same as inexpensive over-the-counter pain relievers.

So, for all the chiropractic hoopla about curing the cause of disease, as far as back pain was concerned, two outcome analyses were finally found that showed that spinal manipulation was no better than a couple of aspirins or Tylenol—and a great deal more expensive, as Dr. Bigos has noted.

The panel's report was published before a Finnish report that basically negated its findings. The Finnish report, as described in Chapter 18 of this book, concluded that doing nothing for acute low back pain was superior to intensive muscle-stretching manipulative procedures.

Dr. Bigos's letter also points out that neck manipulation (which can be risky) was not part of their investigation and also that manipulation was safe only if there were no significant "neurological abnormalities." This, as the guidelines stated, includes sciatica due to a ruptured intervertebral disk; patients with this condition should not undergo manipulation. Ironically, chiropractic claims to be able to adjust vertebrae that supposedly press on nerves, but when confronted with real, demonstrable pressure of a disk on a nerve, causing sciatica, spinal manipulation is both ineffective and unsafe, according to the guidelines.

A third response came from Brian G. Smith, MD, staff orthopedic surgeon for a well-known Connecticut children's center:

> Thank you for your recent correspondence and phone calls regarding your continued efforts in bringing

public awareness to the nature of chiropractic care. Your recent letter to *Connecticut Medicine* was very informative and revealing. In my practice, I still continue to see things that are a nuisance in caring for our patients. Please find enclosed copies of reports on two sisters who recently saw a chiropractic person. I found it quite interesting that "Mary Doe" entered the office with no complaints to accompany her sister but was found to have a "negative alteration in neuromusculature and biomechanical integrity" of her spine and pelvis and then was recommended to have complete radiographs of her spine as well as 3-times-a-week treatment for a period of four weeks. This, again, for a child who was apparently well and simply walked into the office with her sister. Especially, as his own note mentions, when she had no complaints. . . .

The following is the chiropractic report on this patient that we are calling "Mary Doe."

PATIENT REPORT FOR SELECTED PATIENTS

SUBJECTIVE: Mary Doe entered the office with no complaints.

OBJECTIVE:

ROM: Cervical flexion is hypermobile at 60 degrees, extension is normal at 45 degrees, right lateral flexion is normal at 45 degrees, left lateral flexion is decreased to 30 degrees, right rotation is normal at 80 degrees, left rotation is decreased to 60 degrees. Thoracolumbar flexion is normal at 90 degrees, extension is normal at 35 degrees, right lateral flexion is hypermobile at 40 degrees, left lateral flexion is decreased at 30 degrees, right rotation is normal at 30 degrees, left rotation is normal at 30 degrees.

ORTHO:

NEURO:

SOFT TISSUE: There is a negative alteration of the neuromusculature and biomechanical integrity in the cervical, thoracic and lumbosacral spine and pelvis.
ASSESSMENT: Mary is expected to be progressing satisfactorily.
PLAN: The patient will get A-P and lateral full spine radiographs. The patient will receive adjustment of osseous disarticulations, myofascial release and therapeutic hose exercises. The patient will be seen three times weekly to as needed and evaluated in four weeks.

I also received a copy of a letter that a chiropractor had sent to the editor of a publication called *Unique Opportunities*. A medical doctor sent it to me to illustrate how chiropractors overpromote themselves.

Chiropractic not "alternative"

Through my father, who is an MD, I was given the March/April 1997 edition of your magazine. I read with great interest the article "Coming of Age" concerning alternative therapies entering the mainstream. What I found missing in this otherwise well written and balanced piece of reporting concerning "alternative" medicine, is that unlike acupuncture, meditation, homeopathy, herbology, naturopathy, etc., which are types of therapies or "wellness" philosophies, chiropractic medicine is a 102-year-old licensed profession. None of the other types of alternative medicine covered in Ms. Feldman's article are academic disciplines or professions.

The chiropractic profession, like medicine, osteopathy, dentistry, and podiatry, has professionally accredited undergraduate adenopathy graduate programs, with multi-disciplinary faculties, research facilities, and large physical campuses. Chiropractic is a graduate health care profession requiring previous undergraduate studies in the humanities and sciences before a student matriculates in the doctoral program.

Chiropractic is based on scientific principles of anatomy, physiology, and biomechanics of the human body, consistent with allopathic medicine's views of health as "the absence of disease."

Ms. Feldman's definition of alternative health: "focus on optimizing health by strengthening and tuning into the body's own healing abilities" in part defines modern chiropractic care. However, modern chiropractic practice encompasses mainstream health care with a holistic approach.

I find the inclusion of chiropractic with other forms of "alternative medicine" in your article positions it in the category of marginally scientific or unscientific therapies, which are not professions....

Chiropractic embraces scientifically based practice methodology, with a decidedly "hands-on" approach complemented by state-of-the-art diagnostic and testing procedures. Chiropractic stands by itself as a profession, but stresses a holistic approach, which may explain why Ms. Feldman and the physicians she showcases consider my profession "alternative medicine."

The chiropractic profession is far more than simply an alternative type of medicine, but rather a mature profession. It is satisfying that many medical schools, the government, and academic institutions are taking an aggressive approach to studying "alternative medicine." However, I believe chiropractic should be investigated as a profession equal to medicine or dentistry, that has something to contribute to the body of scientific knowledge."

Stephen Barrett, MD, who has investigated chiropractic thoroughly and is editor of this book, has spoken several times with the letter's author and believes that he is medically oriented and practices in a scientific manner. However, the majority of chiropractors do not; the letter's portrayal of chiropractic's status should be regarded as wishful thinking. I also heard from William Mahan, head of the National Health Care Anti-Fraud Association. While not commenting on the validity of chiropractic itself, he noted that chiropractors, as others, can be found guilty of fraud in the real sense. (Chapter 20 provides an example.)

Paul H. Dworkin, MD, editor of the *Journal of Developmental and Behavioral Pediatrics*, also wrote to me:

> Thank you for requesting my views on the success of chiropractic treatment for children with developmental and behavioral problems. . . . We frequently receive manuscripts on a variety of nonstandard therapies for children experiencing developmental and behavioral disorders. Based upon my knowledge of the literature, I am aware of no studies which objectively and scientifically document the value of chiropractic therapy in addressing developmental or behavioral problems. My opinion, based upon my knowledge of the literature, is that any claims of benefit for such therapy among children with developmental and behavioral problems are unwarranted and not based on scientific evidence.
>
> Once again, thank you for soliciting my opinion.
>
> Sincerely yours,
> Paul H. Dworkin, MD

Another letter came from C. Everett Koop, MD, former U.S. Surgeon General, who was kind enough to send his opinions on chiropractic:

> You've taken on a difficult task. Although many people might agree with your general endeavor and the title of your book (Chiropractic, the Greatest Hoax of the Century?), the time for that is probably past. The reason I say this is that now one finds orthodox allopathic

physicians using chiropractors in their practices — not to do what chiropractors claim to do, but as an adjunct to physiotherapy and treatment of low back pain.

I remember the professor of anatomy at Cornell taking a fresh spine out of the cadaver and trying to subluxate anything — of course, he couldn't.

I wish you well, however you decide to go, but I know it's an uphill fight.

> Sincerely yours,
> C. Everett Koop, MD

Another opinion came from Paul Shekelle, MD, PhD, who headed the famous Rand study on which the AHCPR guidelines were largely based. He was helpful in sending me a package of his studies and the following letter from Rand, where he is employed:

Thank you for your interest in our work. I am enclosing the reprints you requested plus other related materials.

RAND's work on spinal manipulation has been funded by two private foundations associated with chiropractors and by the Agency for Health Care Policy and Research, a branch of the United States Public Health Service.

The optimum management for low back pain continues to be a question for ongoing research. Some observational studies, such as the Carey Study, in the *New England Journal of Medicine* to which you refer, show no difference among groups. Some experimental studies show a benefit from manipulation, others do not. The net weight of the evidence for acute low back pain continues to be positive in favor of manipulation.

> Sincerely,
> Paul Shekelle, MD, PhD

Shekelle's candid statement adds to the evidence that the AHCPR study was not an endorsement of chiropractic. In reviewing the complex statistical analysis on which the Rand meta-analysis was based, I find no mention of "adjustments" of vertebral "subluxation" or spinal misalignments, only spinal manipulation. Moreover, the cited research did not include attempts to find the cause of low back pain or just what spinal manipulations were supposed to accomplish. Dr. Shekelle is certainly correct in saying the optimum management of low back pain continues to be a question of ongoing research.

Another interesting letter came from Ira C. Magaziner, who was chief advisor to Hilary Clinton in her ill-fated health care reform proposal and President Clinton's senior advisor for policy development. I had met Magaziner at a town hall meeting in Manchester, Connecticut, arranged by Congresswoman Barbara Kennelley. I impressed upon him my concerns about the inroads being made by unscientific "alternative" health care, including chiropractic. Describing how these reminded me of the snake oil medicine men of the 1800s, I also stated that reform was long overdue. In response, he sent the following letter.

Thank you for sharing your thoughts about health care reform. You expressed concern about chiropractic care under the President's Health Care Reform Proposal. This is an issue the Administration considered carefully while formulating the proposal.

The President's proposal provides coverage for a comprehensive benefit package, including services of health professionals. The proposal defines health professional services to include those services which are lawfully provided by a physician, or those services that could be performed by a physician and that are provided by another person who is legally authorized to provide those services in the state. The proposal does not specify particular items or services within these broad categories, nor does it identify specific providers of services. Improved competition among health plans may create new incentives for effective use of a range of providers, including chiropractors. Plans will be free to use any mix of providers to meet the needs of their enrollees.

This nation now has a historic opportunity to change our health care system to make it work for all of us. I hope you will work with the President to make health security a reality for all Americans.
Regards,
Ira C. Magaziner

Magaziner took the politically "safe" ground that where anyone is licensed to provide any kind of health care, the president would support it. I believe that the proliferation of worthless, unscientific, unproven health care provides no health security and would waste much-needed health care dollars. Fixing this problem, I related to him, would be real health care reform.

Arnold S. Relman, MD, editor-in-chief emeritus of the prestigious *New England Journal of Medicine*, gave this opinion:

I have not been following chiropractic "research" for several years, but I am not aware of any studies published in the medical literature that relate to the "subluxation" theory upon which chiropractors base their therapy. There have been one or two studies, which I assume you are aware, that compare the symptomatic relief of nonspecific low back pain by chiropractic therapy with that produced by conventional conservative medical management. These studies have shown that chiropractic manipulation produces at least as much symptomatic relief as conventional medical treatment. Aside from this work, I know no other credible clinical study of chiropractic treatment that has been published in the peer reviewed medical literature. However, I must repeat the caveat that I really haven't followed the field closely and may, therefore, have missed some significant literature.
Sincerely yours,
Arnold S. Relman, MD

In a 1979 editorial, Dr. Relman had challenged chiropractors to prove scientifically the existence of vertebral "subluxations" or abandon the chiropractic theory. No such studies exist.

Mention was previously made of the opinions of chiropractor Louis Sportelli of Palmerton, Pennsylvania, a spokesman for chiropractic and former board chairman of the American Chiropractic Association (ACA), who, after my visit to New York Chiropractic College, had sent me a detailed three-page letter along with a package of chiropractic literature that included Dr. Scott Haldeman's textbook. Sportelli's letter, typical of present-day chiropractic strategy, criticized medical care and praised chiropractic. He stated:

> The underlying fact which is about to emerge from all of the outcomes research is simply this — most medical health care decisions are arbitrary and harmful to patients. This is the sad state of medical care in this country today. . . . Only about 1% of the articles in medical journals are scientifically sound.

The book *Chiropractic: The Victim's Perspective* quotes Sportelli as saying, "We're the only profession that can do something in a patient to insure wellness before they get sick. I get adjusted every week, and I have for the past 35 years of my life." This book was written by the late George Magner, with a forward by William G. Jarvis, PhD, president of the National Council Against Health Fraud. Magner characterized subluxation theory and its trappings as "a delusional system—a set of beliefs held despite abundant evidence that contradicts them" and observed that "as things stand now, chiropractic is clinging for dear life to its cultist and pseudoscientific roots while insisting that it has risen above them." These statements are commendable and in keeping with my own conclusions.

Finally, I sent a questionnaire to all American and Canadian medical school deans and more editors of scientific journals asking whether, in their opinion, the chiropractic theory was "true" or "false." Of the 27 deans who replied, all said that it was false.

Dr. George M. Lundberg, then-editor of the *Journal of the American Medical Association*, agreed that the theory was "false." He also remarked that the term "neural integrity" used by the chiropractic deans was unclear and that the phrase "may influence organ system function" was meaningless. He summarized his opinion with the statement, "No scientific basis for this theory as a cause of organ system health or disease."

Dr. Jerold T. Lucy, editor of *Pediatrics*, replied less diplomatically, "It's garbage!"

Dr. James Dolin, editor of the *Archives of Medicine*, and Dr. J. Claude Bennett, editor of *The Journal of Medicine*, both replied, "false."

I received the following letter from Dr. William Harlan, then-acting director of the National Center for Complementary and Alternative Medicine:

> Your letter to Donna Shalala, Secretary of the Department of Health and Human Services, was forwarded to the National Institutes of Health (NIH) National Center for Complementary and Alternative Medicine (NCCAM) for response. . . . Your statement that "this is long overdue . . . for your administration to assess again chiropractic," is one that is timely.
>
> The NIH recently established the NCCAM to conduct evaluations of chiropractic and alternative therapies. As stated succinctly by Dr Harold Varmus, the Director of NIH, in his speech at the Stamford University Medical School Graduation ceremony, "There are methods that work and methods that don't. Or methods that have been tested and those that have not." It is the ultimate goal of NIH and NCCAM to develop and fund research that will clearly, unambiguously, and definitely show which therapies commonly referred to as "Alternative" are effective and safe. Chiropractic medicine is included in the group of alternative treatments currently

being investigated. NIH and NCCAM will disseminate
the results of this research when they are available.

Thank you for your comments on chiropractic, and
we agree that further evaluation is needed.

The bottom line, supported by most of the responses
described in this chapter, is that chiropractic's "subluxation
theory" is a hoax.

14
Reactions to the First Edition of This Book

Following publication of this book's first edition, there were several revealing reviews and reactions. Major reviews were made by the American Chiropractic Association (ACA) and the Connecticut Chiropractic Association (CCA), and one appeared in *Connecticut Medicine*, the journal of the Connecticut State Medical Society.

My basic response to the ACA review is the same as stated in Chapter 10 (Visits to Two Chiropractic Colleges). There is no scientific evidence for the chiropractic theory that (a) vertebral "subluxations" press on nerves, interfering with passage of energy to various organs, and thereby causing disease, and (b) spinal "adjustments" of those mythical entities can prevent, effectively treat, or cure any disease. Here is the ACA review, with my responses interspersed:

> While the American Chiropractic Association respects open dialogue on the subject of chiropractic care, we view *Chiropractic: The Greatest Hoax of the Century?* as a biased, misinformed treatment of one of the most popular and effective forms of health care available today.

My response: Chiropractic has been misinforming the public for more than 100 years and is challenged by my book to prove the validity of its claims. Popular trends do not validate a practice. Popular smoking, overeating, and illicit drug use do not make them healthy practices.

Chiropractic care is validated by a number of research studies. The 1994 US Agency for Health Care Policy and Research [AHCPR] panel concluded that spinal manipulation is a recommended form of initial treatment for low back pain in adults. The prestigious Rand Corporation also determined that spinal manipulation is an appropriate treatment for acute low back pain, and reported from its analysis that 94 percent of all manipulations are performed by doctors of chiropractic.

My response: The book's last chapter contained an editorial by Dr. Paul Shekelle, chief investigator for the Rand report, stating that, "It is currently inappropriate to consider chiropractic as a broad based alternative to traditional care." In a letter to me, he stated, "The optimum management for low back pain continues to be a question for ongoing research." Also, the letter from Dr. Stanley Bigos, chairman of the AHCPR panel, places the AHCPR guidelines in perspective. There is no mention of chiropractic, "subluxations," or "adjustments" in the entire report.

Chiropractic is one of the safest forms of health care available today. According to another study by the Rand Corporation, a serious adverse reaction from cervical manipulation—or manipulation of the neck—occurs one in a million manipulations. The same Rand study showed that, on extremely rare occasions that when an adverse reaction does occur, it is the result of improperly trained physical therapists or other health care providers, not chiropractors performing this procedure.

My response: There are no clear figures as to just how many strokes and how much damage to the vertebral arteries occur every year from cervical manipulations, but there are probably at least 100 strokes a year. Since there are few sensible indications for neck manipulations for any condition in the first place, any catastrophic tragedy from such manipulation is unconscionable. What damage this may be doing to newborn children, allegedly to prevent SID syndrome, is unknown. My report on

Linda Solsbury (Chapter 9 in this edition of my book) describes how she was paralyzed by chiropractic neck manipulation and subsequently received a $10 million malpractice jury award.

> In contrast, a study published in the April 15, 1998, issue of the *Journal of the American Medical Association* found that more than 2 million Americans become seriously ill every year from reactions to correctly prescribed drugs and 106,000 die from these side effects.

My response: These figures have been challenged. It is admitted that many drugs such as those used for AIDS and cancer treatment do have a high risk/benefit ratio. The side effects are well described and not hidden. The real harm of chiropractic is in inadequate diagnosis and in completely ineffective treatment for any disease, since the chiropractic belief is that the cause of all disease is the theoretical nonexistent vertebral "subluxation," and the primary treatment is spinal "adjustment."

> Dr. Chotkowski's mission to defeat chiropractic is not embraced by the medical community. In fact, the Sept. 2, 1998 issue of the *JAMA* reports that a number of U.S. medical schools are offering courses teaching students to work with patients who need or want to be treated by alternative health care providers such as doctors of chiropractic. In addition, the November 11 issue of *JAMA* reports that 4 out of 10 Americans used at least one form of alternative care in 1997, with 90 percent receiving chiropractic care."

My response: Twenty-seven medical deans surveyed agreed with me that the chiropractic theory and practice based on it is false. I feel that, as a person dedicated to the scientific method of treating health conditions of life and death, I have a moral, professional obligation to inform the public of the total truth about chiropractic care. My book lays down the challenge to chiropractic to prove their claims with scientific evidence, which they have yet been unable to do in more than 100 years.

Finally, more than 20 million Americans seek chiropractic care each year and, according to a Gallup survey, 90
percent of them say their care was effective. We feel
these patients would agree that Dr. Chotkowski's attack
is unfounded and that the book does a grave disservice
to a community of people making informed health care
decisions based on research and successful outcomes.

My response: The claim, if true, that more than 20 million Americans seek out this false method of health care only compounds
the enormity of the hoax. My book is not an "attack" against
chiropractic. It is an exposé of a gigantic hoax. The hoax thesis
is well documented and supported with scientific evidence and
by opinions of members of the scientific community. Thus, the
book is hopefully a service to humanity.

Connecticut Medicine offered this review.

The overwhelming theme, (of the book) is that . . . the
burden of scientific proof of effectiveness of chiropractic treatment has been thrust upon chiropractic for the
past century. This chiropractic has failed to do as chiropractic itself admits.

The book, like chiropractic itself, relies on newspaper articles, author research (3 decades of primary care),
and anecdotes to weave a story of concern. With the
number of licensed chiropractors growing to 69,000 in
1997, the author defines the problem, reduces the issues and clearly pronounces a solution. He insists that
chiropractic schools, as osteopathic schools before them,
"Convert their colleges into standard medical schools."

With persistence to detail, he reviews the eight-mem-
ber panel's recommendation to then-Secretary of H.E.W.
Wilbur Cohen in the early 1970s, noting that although
chiropractic was accepted into Medicare provider status, the panel judged negatively because:

a. Chiropractic knowledge is not consistent with adequate scientific research.
b. Subluxation is not a significant factor in the disease process; spinal analysis and the adjustments are thus not fruitful.
c. Manipulation must be studied through suitable scientific research.
d. Inadequacies of chiropractic education and the deemphasis of proven causative factors and disease processes make it unlikely that an adequate diagnosis or treatment plan is possible.

There is a short visit to New York Chiropractic College and a review of the *Principles and Practices of Chiropractic*, the book known as the "Bible."

The author addresses the issues of risk management and concludes with the ominous note that, "the chiropractic profession has existed for a century without having made a single contribution to the world's knowledge in the health sciences." However, an addendum does note that a Canadian chiropractic college studied asthma and spinal manipulation, and no benefit was found. The second study from Seattle and Edmonton also concluded that chiropractic manipulation for low back pain was only marginally better than the minimal intervention of a simple education booklet."

I believe that Dr. Chotkowski has successfully approached and defined the chiropractic arena medically, legally, congressionally, and personally.

A contrary review came from CCA president Brian Baker, DC:

On behalf of the Connecticut Chiropractic Association I would like to respond to the book review of L.A. Chotkowski's self-published book, *Chiropractic: The Greatest Hoax of the Century?*, that was published in your November issue.

That your reviewer, C. Robert Biondino, gave this book a favorable review is baffling. Chotkowski's comments and sweeping condemnation of chiropractic are based on nothing but (as Biondino acknowledges) "newspaper articles, author research (three decades of primary practice), and anecdotes." Hardly sound, evidenced based, science and research.

The fact is Chotkowski has publicly made it his life's work to vilify chiropractic. That his book was self-published through New England Novelty Books alone should cast some light on his "objectivity." What your reviewer failed to do was disclose this bias and critically evaluate Chotkowski's statements.

Unfortunately Dr. Chotkowski steadfastly refuses to acknowledge published research favorable toward chiropractic. Two recent examples of research analysis are the Agency for Health Care Policy research review of studies and support of spinal manipulation for low back pain, and the Ontario Ministry of Health's published report reviewing Chiropractic research and literature with a final recommendation for increased utilization of chiropractic in their health-care service.

The chiropractic profession has taken its responsibility continually to produce research and evidence seriously. It has only been recently that barriers have been overcome and increased governmental funding been provided.

What is truly remarkable is the volume of research that the profession produced before having access to national and governmental funding sources like NIH. Chotkowski and your reviewer appear oblivious to this information.

Chotkowski's opinion that "The chiropractic profession has existed for a century without having made a single notable contribution to the world's body of knowledge in the health sciences" is as absurd as it sounds. When your reviewer writes "Chotkowski has successfully approached and defined the chiropractic arena medically, legally, congressionally, and personally," he should have added that Chotkowski failed to do so credibly. The Connecticut Chiropractic Association makes efforts to reach out to the medical community to share information on chiropractic procedure and practice. When CSMS gives this type of book a forum and implied credibility, many of us ask: "Why bother?"

My response to Baker was succinct and to the point as reported in *Connecticut Medicine*, as follows:

Chiropractor Brian Baker, president of the Connecticut Chiropractic Association, writing in its behalf, in his response to a review of my book by Dr. C. Robert Biondino, has erroneously stated that the book *Chiropractic: The Greatest Hoax of the Century?* did not acknowledge the research findings on acute low back pain by the Agency for Health Care Policy and Research. The book contains an entire chapter devoted to that subject.

In addition, the book goes one step further in containing personal communications from the chairman of that AHCPR panel Dr. Stanley Bigos, Professor of Orthopedics and Environmental Health, University of Washington Medical School, and a second letter from Dr. Paul Shekelle, chief investigator for the chiropractic-funded Rand Corp. study on which the AHCPR findings were primarily based.

Furthermore, the book reports the most recent findings that chiropractic spinal adjustments are of little value in the treatment of low back pain.

The basic thrust of the book remains unchallenged by chiropractor Baker. Despite the passage of over a hundred years, chiropractic has failed to prove its theory of "vertebral subluxations" pressing on nerves causing disease, or that spinal "adjustments" are effective treatment for any disease.

Chiropractor Baker has attempted to obfuscate the issue by accusing the author of the book of "bias and lack of objectivity." The fact is that 27 medical college deans who responded to my survey, unanimously agreed with me that the theory and practice of chiropractic was false. Scientific medical authorities like Dr. C. Everett Koop, former U.S. Surgeon General, Dr. George Lundberg, then-editor of the *Journal of the AMA*, Dr. Paul Dworkin, editor of the journal *Developmental and Behavioral Pediatrics*, Dr. Arnold Relman, editor emeritus of the *New England Journal of Medicine*, and a host of others, whose personal letters support my findings, are all in the book.

Finally, chiropractor Baker has failed in his review to indicate just what contribution chiropractic has made to scientific health care over the past century. In essence he has failed to negate the book's conclusion that chiropractic has made none, and that the theory and practice of chiropractic is a false hoax as documented.

Louis Sportelli, DC, a major spokesman for chiropractic, who claims his regular spinal "adjustments" have maintained his health for years, offered some additional choice remarks:

I have read your book and find you to be beyond bias. You and your ilk are so out of touch with reality that you cannot realize the world has passed you by. You assume that chiropractic is engaged in unscientific medicine and yet you remain silent as the epidemic of medical errors runs rampant. You will see that the notion that medicine is scientific is becoming more ludicrous each day. Look to your own "glass house."

My response: Medical "bias" and "errors" are two major defense themes frequently used by chiropractic, and Sportelli uses them quite enthusiastically. It is medieval chiropractic that has been passed by with modern medicine.

More than 50 brief reviews of the book were posted to the Amazon and Barnes & Noble Web sites. Many of these revealed chiropractic's frustration over the book's challenge. Most were written by chiropractors or their true-believer patients. Here are some excerpts:

* * *

The book makes a solid point that the basic theory of chiropractic is utter nonsense. Despite a hundred years of existence, chiropractic has not demonstrated the existence of the "subluxation" much less that it causes disease (or "dis-ease") or that chiropractic methods can identify such lesions and correct them.

* * *

Don't even bother to read this book. I purchased it before going to a chiropractor and was scared stiff.

* * *

"Scientific" medicine is the third leading cause of death in the US. Enough said.

* * *

More than identifying it as a hoax, a solution is offered!! ... This philosophy is about as unproven as alien visitors.

* * *

Chiropractors usually are far superior to MD's!!! This book is a farce and is representative of the closed-mindedness of too many MDs.

* * *

Excellent book. Public needs to be aware that chiropractic is voodoo medicine.

* * *

A chiropractor saved me from back surgery. My daughter had asthma for the first 11 years of her life. After a course of chiropractic care, her symptoms went away.

* * *

Anecdotal accounts do not determine what is true.

* * *

A beautiful art, falsely attacked again. Tears built up in my eyes.

* * *

Man who is on thin ice should jump. After reading this book I had to laugh.

* * *

Books like this show how ignorant the medical profession is about chiropractic.

* * *

Sickening. The AMA propaganda against chiropractors is alive and well. I feel inspired to write a book about how modern medicine is the most destructive force in our society and itself may be the most colossal hoax of all time.

* * *

On the positive side, one reader stated, "Dr. Chotkowski's attempt should be applauded in light of the ever-growing and unfortunate power of chiropractors." Another quipped, "The emperor has no clothes (or subluxation)." And another said, "Everyone should read this book before considering chiropractic treatment."

The word "cult" has been criticized when applied to chiropractic, yet the language of my critics indicates levels of belief and devotion typical of cult members.

15
More Dialogue and Debate
on the Internet

Hoping to become better acquainted with the feelings of the chiropractic community on the "philosophy" of chiropractic, I engaged in a dialogue-debate with chiropractors on various Web sites on the Internet.

* * *

One of the first responses came gratuitously from Dynamic Chiropractic Online. Titled "The War's Over, But MD Continues the Fight," it stated:

> On March 10, 1974 on the island of Lubang in a remote part of the Philippine archipelago, Second Lieutenant Hiroo Oneda of the Japanese Imperial Army was ordered to surrender by his commanding officer, Major Taniguchi, after 30 years.
>
> Reminiscent of poor Hiro, although less dramatic, is L.A.Chotkowski, MD, who on August 26, 1997 sent this memo to the "scientific community." [As noted in Chapter 13 of this book, the memo asked for opinions about the chiropractic theory of subluxations and adjustments.] The responses to Dr. Chotkowski's appeal criticizing chiropractic were predictable.
>
> Had Dr. Chotkowski seriously considered Dr. David Eisenberg's most recent study of "alternative medicine" use in the U.S., he would have discovered that the number of visits to "alternative care providers" in 1997 was nearly double the number of visits to all "primary care physicians." Perhaps someone can get through to Dr. Chotkowski. The war is over.

I responded:

> The war may be over but the question raised in my book remains unresolved for over a hundred years. The question not addressed by Dynamic is whether there is such an entity as a vertebral subluxation causing disease? Furthermore, clear evidence is lacking anywhere that chiropractic can prevent, effectively treat, or cure any single disease.

> It is clear from this exchange that chiropractic fears confrontation and exposé and would like very much to be accepted by the scientific community.

> As for the finding in the Eisenberg study that large numbers of people seek "unscientific alternative care," this only corroborates the enormity of the chiropractic hoax in my view.

* * *

Anthony Rosner, PhD, executive director of the Federation for Chiropractic Education and Research, reviewed my book on his organization's Web site. His criticisms were referenced with a long list of reports supposedly validating his views. However, nothing that he said refuted the book's basic thesis that subluxation theory is false.

* * *

Nearly every day for about about 5 months, on a chiropractic forum called Hot Topics, there were messages between chiropractors and myself and between chiropractors and themselves, in perhaps one of the most remarkable medical doctor-chiropractic dialogues ever. I was originally welcomed, but after I posed a list of embarrassing, challenging questions, the host decided to limit participation to chiropractors only.

Some of the most interesting posts came from chiropractic students who questioned the validity of their theory and practice and asked whether they were being misled into believing they were prepared to deal with disease like "real" doctors. One former student reported:

Dr Chot. [my email name], I commend you for taking a stand on chiropractic!

I started Chiro school not knowing what to expect. A couple of weeks into school I was recruited by a student to enter my college's student clinic. I was subjected to full body X-rays when I wasn't experiencing any symptoms. I was then given a sales pitch the intern had memorized that chiropractic could help my back "problem." My intern then treated me for a whole trimester. I repeatedly told him I had absolutely no pain, yet he still adjusted me anyway. He told me that he's recruited a few patients, but if he gets desperate, he'll recruit his sister and her husband.

What did I learn in Chiro college? I learned that a vast majority of smart people can be easily duped by such a scam. I only wasted one trimester of my life and money there. I am currently applying to Med. school. I would rather take my chances of not getting into medical school than to stay in a profession that is a lie.

Posted by Future MD

* * *

The American Chiropractic Association (ACA) submitted a message on chiropractic education to this Hot Topics forum, which stated, in part:

Doctors of chiropractic (DCs), who are licensed to practice in all 50 states and in many nations around the world, undergo rigorous education in the healing sciences, similar to that of medical physicians. In some areas such as anatomy, physiology, rehabilitation, nutrition and public health, they receive more intensive education than their MD counterparts.

However, several students posted messages stating that much of their time was spent listening to indoctrinating lectures on the "philosophy" of chiropractic. After 2 years or so of basic science courses, most student time is spent in manipulating spines in DC offices or clinics. At no time is there any exposure or training in a hospital diagnosing and treating medically ill people, as medical doctors typically do for at least 6 years. Chiropractic students are required to perform a minimum number of "adjustments" before graduation and often must resort to recruiting anyone for that purpose.

The lack of adequate clinical exposure was acknowledged by a chiropractor who stated, "Our schools do not promote problem-based clinical exposure to real people with real problems. Our clinical experience is all about numbers, not learning."

* * *

In order to determine the attitude of practicing chiropractors about the issue of "subluxations," I posed the following challenging questions. "What exactly is a subluxation, and do you believe it exists?" One of the first chiropractors to respond stated: "Let's define subluxation. Choose a model with it's components. Whether it be the five-component model (i.e. spinokinesiology, neuropathology, etc.) or the newer model three-phase (dysautonomia), just pick a model." A second definition came from the ACA:

> By definition, subluxation is a slight dislocation or biomechanical malfunctioning of the vertebrae. Chiropractors often refer to the misalignment of the vertebrae as subluxation. Doctors are trained to restore misaligned vertebrae to their proper position in the spinal cord through a procedure called "spinal adjustment" or "manipulation."

From a disbelieving chiropractor: "Dr Chotkowski is right. I'll have plenty of referrals while you 'SUBLUXATION REMOVERS' are out their brainwashing the public."

Another chiropractor: "Ah, the dreaded subluxation, the silent killer that we chiropractic missionaries are all on a world wide quest to eliminate. Our philosophy regarding Subluxations is seriously outdated and in many ways, ridiculous."

Still another: "But as long as we pray to our Innate as god, this medical nazi will have plenty of fuel to keep his fire going."

From someone calling himself a critical thinker: "You expect anyone on this board to answer a direct, unambigous question regarding the central tenet of chiropractic——our very reason for being? Don't hold your breath."

From a chiropractor named "Spinedoc": "Sorry fellow chiropractors, but it's time to hang up the chiropractic dogma of subluxation. We should not define our scope of practice as manipulation, rather we should define our scope as managers of somatic dysfunction."

And from an evidently very frustrated chiropractor: "I have noticed several messages with the heading 'Chot for brains.' I know this is implying shit for brains and I think we should stop because we are giving shit a bad name."

Objecting to this language, another chiropractor stated:

I have read all the posts in this interesting debate brought about by Dr. Chot and am appalled by the conduct of some of the chiropractors. Yet I have not read one unseemingly attack from him. Indeed throughout this onslaught he has maintained his dignity and professionalism by responding with class, substance, and not being hijacked with emotion.

He has presented a strong argument and is obviously very intelligent and well learned in medicine and science. Can you imagine Dr Chot being referenced in future texts on philosophy and history as the 'reconstructor' of chiropractic.

* * *

There is no question that much dissension exists among chiropractors about "subluxations." However, these mythical entities are not likely to be abandoned—for without them, chiropractic would lose its claim to being a "separate and distinct profession." On the related subject of "adjustments," a Dr. P. pretty well summarized the dilemma. He posted:

What is an adjustment? I feel that delegates from the ACA and ICA and chiropractic college presidents should meet once every year to evaluate new techniques. I have seen weird techniques done by chiropractors. We need a strong leadership that can stand up and proclaim what chiropractic is and what it is not. Physical therapists will one day be able to manipulate in all 50 states

* * *

The healthfraud discusslist, another forum in which I participate, held a similar debate about chiropractic. After much discussion, I proposed a series of 10 satirical commandments for chiropractic behavior.

Thou shalt convince all patients to believe.

Thou shalt praise all you do as natural, beneficial, and compassionate.

Thou shalt condemn all medical science does as unnatural, harmful, and selfish.

Thou shalt accuse the pharmaceutical establishment of a scurrilous vendetta.

Thou shalt declare all medical drugs as poisonous and to be avoided at all costs.

Thou shalt sell supplementary vitamins, herbs, and minerals as nutritional cure-alls.

Thou shalt indoctrinate a fear of surgery and of immunization in children.

Thou shalt accuse doctors of being lackeys of the AMA in a giant conspiracy against you, for their own selfish economic greed.

Thou shalt promote x-rays of the spine to demonstrate subluxations anywhere you desire them to be.

Thou shalt brainwash all patients into believing your adjustments are vital to their health—from the cradle to the grave.

An acerbic reply came from an angry chiropractor: "Thou art an asshole."

My not-so-nice reply: "Any intelligent response challenging the commandments is awaited, but it will surely be a freezing day in hell before that happens."

* * *

When the issue of chiropractic pediatrics was raised, I stated that treating a child with spinal manipulations for acute asthma, ear infections, etc., was tantamount to child abuse.

A study of the pediatric practice of 150 chiropractors in the Boston area was posted in this debate. The report had appeared in the *Archives of Pediatrics*, an American Medical Association publication. The results were as follows:

Respondents had an average 122 patient visits weekly, of which 13 (11%) were children and adolescents. Average visit fees were $82 initial and $38 follow-up, and 49% were covered by insurance. Seventy percent of the respondents recommended herbs and dietary supplements. For pediatric care, 30% reported recommending childhood immunizations. Presented with a hypothetical 2 week old neonate with fever, 17% would treat the patient themselves rather than immediately refer the patient to a doctor of medicine or emergency facility.

The report concluded that "children and adolescents constitute a substantial number of patients in chiropractics. An estimated 420,000 pediatric visits were made in the Boston Metropolitan area in 1998, costing approximately $14 million. Pediatric chiropractic care is often inconsistent with recommended guidelines. National studies are needed to assess safety, efficacy, and cost of chiropractic care for children."

The journal's editor, Catherine D. DeAngelis, MD, commented that, "When I contemplate a chiropractor treating a 2 week-old neonate with fever, I get a gigantic backache."

* * *

The last contribution to this dialogue came fittingly from Walter I. Wardwell, PhD, professor emeritus of sociology,

University of Connecticut, and a leading chiropractic historian and proponent. In the "DC Archives" section of the chiropractic Web site called Chiroweb, he commented on the lack of unity in chiropractic beliefs and practices:

> In this my final publication, I take the opportunity to strongly recommend to the chiropractic profession in America that it do what has been proposed over most of its history by many others, including most of the leaders of the profession. The disparate segments of the profession should give up their minor differences and merge into one strong national association. Wake up and see the light. Unite and begin to reap the benefits.

* * *

I have tried to choose significant excerpts from the hundreds of opinions about chiropractic posted to Internet news groups and Web sites. Most are direct quotations, but since they are necessarily excerpts, their complete impact is sometimes diminished. However, they clearly reflect the fact that chiropractors cannot agree among themselves about the nature or significance of "subluxations."

Chiropractors also differ about their scope and treatment methods. Some limit their practice to manipulation of muscles and joints only for musculoskeletal conditions, whereas others purport to treat a wide variety of problems. Some stick with manipulation and/or physical therapy techniques, whereas others dabble in dubious dietary supplements, homeopathy, herbology, acupuncture, and/or whatever else strikes their fancy or lines their pocketbooks.

Overall, this dialogue-debate presented no plausible evidence that the chiropractic notions of "subluxations" and "adjustments" and their associated practices are other than a hoax.

Part IV

Additional Perspectives

16
Why People Go
to Chiropractors

During my medical practice, there was ample opportunity to observe why people visit chiropractors. One reason is the inability of standard medical care to cure or relieve all diseases. Many years ago, before polio was wiped out with medical science's vaccine, it was one of the major diseases that chiropractors claimed to cure. They have also claimed to be able to treat multiple sclerosis. This is an ideal disease for making quack claims because its natural course usually includes remissions and exacerbations and any improvement could be attributed to spinal manipulation or whatever else a chiropractor wanted to do. The Spears Clinic, a now-defunct chiropractic hospital, used to send me solicitations picturing how multiple sclerosis patients entered the clinic in a wheelchair and walked out with great smiles.

Another source of dissatisfaction with medical care is that it often requires taking medications that have adverse effects. Those for high blood pressure, for example, can cause impotence and interfere dramatically with patients' lifestyles. Even aspirin, perhaps the most commonly used drug of all, can have undesirable side effects. It is not surprising that the promise of drugless treatment is so appealing—but potentially tragic in the long run.

Many patients go to chiropractors because they fear surgery, particularly brain and heart surgery for which the fatality rates are relatively high. Patients with a potentially fatal disease like cancer may seek an "alternative" to avoid the discomfort of radiation or chemotherapy. Twisting the spine to allegedly enhance the immune system might be a "straw" that a desperately ill patient may "grasp."

Another reason for resorting to chiropractic is a failure to understand the difference between scientific medicine and unscientific chiropractic. Although chiropractors have failed to demonstrate their alleged "subluxations," many of them use weasel-worded descriptions to make themselves more believable.

Chiropractors cleverly play the "bash-the-American Medical Association and bash-the-doctor game" by claiming that doctors who criticize them are merely afraid of competition. The federal judge who ruled in the chiropractic antitrust suit against the AMA concluded that the AMA had attacked chiropractic in an attempt to protect the public and not for economic reasons (see Chapter 17). Yet economic ploys have credibility to many people who distrust doctors or medical science.

Despite the enormous amount of scientific progress in health matters, many people still have little knowledge of health and disease and are unable to judge between proven factual health knowledge and phony claims. Many books promote all sorts of ludicrous claims made for various types of "alternative" health care. There are books on miracle diets and miracle cures for just about every health problem known to medical science. People seeking help for a serious disease are often misled by false claims and promises. How else could the parents of a child with a neck tumor exposéd on the ABC-TV's "20/20" program feel that a chiropractor could cure the tumor by twisting the child's neck? Even though this resulted in the child's paralysis, the family returned for further neck manipulation.

Highly Questionable Salesmanship

Subluxation-based chiropractic is basically a belief system with "principles" that cannot be demonstrated by scientific means. Once a belief is implanted into the human mind, there is no need for reason or proof.

Many chiropractors sell themselves through newspaper advertisements, television infomercials, and lectures. For years, the AMA and the medical profession believed it was unethical to advertise and that a doctor's reputation and professional skills rather than advertising hype should be what counts. Now, it seems that everyone in the health care field advertises—insurance companies, medical doctors, hospitals, health spas, naturopaths, chiropractors, and anyone related to health care. But chiropractors probably promote themselves more elaborately than any of the others.

Chiropractic promises health care "the natural way" with "adjustments" and manipulations, without mentioning the harmful effects of these procedures. Just what this word "natural" is supposed to mean is not clear, particularly as related to chiropractic. "Natural" is a buzzword, presumably for harmless, pristine, unpolluted, nonsynthetic health. This, by definition, presumably excludes the use of medicines or surgery which, according to chiropractic, are dangerous. This type of advertising can discourage patients from seeking the benefits of modern medicine.

Some advertisements include nutrition and what are called diagnostic services. How a chiropractor can claim ability to diagnose disease without any experience with or exposure to diseases in a general hospital goes unanswered. Medical doctors, by contrast, after intensive study of hundreds of diseases for 4 years, generally spend several more years of specialty training in which they deal with patients, mainly at hospitals.

Many chiropractors still claim to treat the "cause" of disease and criticize the medical profession for "only treating symptoms." The exact opposite is actually the case. Chiropractors basically treat pain, whatever the cause. The idea that "subluxations" cause disease has been debunked by medical science, as discussed in this book and elsewhere. While twisting backs and necks for more than 100 years, chiropractors have contributed nothing to medical science.

For years, chiropractors have emphasized practice-building. In the book *At Your Own Risk,* the author, Ralph Lee Smith, describes how the Parker School of Professional Services "seems to be nothing less than turning the entire chiropractic profession into an army of smooth-talking, wheeling and dealing supersalesmen, engaged in a gigantic con artist game." Smith attended one of its seminars posing as a chiropractor and joining 200 others. He reported how chiropractors were taught how to (a) frighten patients away from medical doctors; (b) give free consultations; (c) concentrate on the spine as the cause of a patient's problems; (d) lather the patients with love; (e) emphasize their condition as chronic and requiring long-term care; and (f) build fear that the patient's condition could be serious, but that natural chiropractic can work wonders. Smith summed up the seminar's teaching's this way:

> Throughout the procedure the chiropractor tries to wean the patient away from established medical treatment— permanently, if possible. "A true chiropractic patient," says the *Textbook*, "is one whose convictions with regard to health have been diverted from the muddy road of medicine to the superhighway of chiropractic by a series of correlated mental concepts, positively implanted in proper order."

Part of the fear strategy is to emphasize dangers of drug side effects and surgery as opposed to "natural healing" measures supposedly provided by adjustments. Of course, some people go to chiropractors because they "just don't like doctors."

Chiropractors are licensed. The public tends to regard licensing as evidence of legitimacy, but chiropractic licensing was accomplished by persistent lobbying rather than by proof of validity. Medicines must pass strict Food and Drug Administration standards for safety and effectiveness before approval. On the other hand, chiropractic licensure was based on political rather than scientific activity.

Chiropractors advertise that their services are covered by insurance companies and Medicare. Many states require insurance companies to carry some form of chiropractic coverage. The 1972 Medicare law authorized payment only in cases in which a "subluxation" was supposedly demonstrated by x-ray. Since chiropractic "subluxations" are not actually visible on x-ray films, this should have prevented Medicare payments to chiropractors. However, this requirement was not strictly enforced and was abolished on January 1, 2000, after it became apparent that it was senseless.

Some chiropractors make claims through patient testimonials. I have seen long lines of patients testifying at legislative hearings in Connecticut about the alleged benefits they have received from chiropractic "adjustments." Although this type of evidence is very effective when used politically, it is not scientific proof. Chiropractic has relied on this type of evidence, either anecdotal or in outcome studies, rather than on any basic scientific research into the nature of "subluxations" and "adjustments."

Chiropractic advertises that it "helps children develop into healthy adults." Parents are being advised to consider a chiropractor even before the child is born. A chiropractic publication called *Spinal Column* contains a full-page spread titled "Chiropractic Care: A Total Wellness Plan for the Whole Family," which states:

> One of the first subluxations experienced is during the birth process. As the child grows and becomes more active, he can experience spinal misalignments from normal play activities and falls. It is important to have your child's spine checked on a regular basis. This will help insure proper development and the best possible health.

In contrast, Ronald Slaughter, DC, president of the National Association for Chiropractic Medicine, warns that no child younger than 12 years should ever be taken to a chiropractor unless recommended by a pediatrician because children's bone structures are still developing and manipulation can cause damage.

Here in Connecticut, a television infomercial showed a chiropractor manipulating the back of a newborn and stating, "As the twig is bent, so grows the tree." Parker Professional Products, one of the largest practice-building suppliers, sells a poster with the same message, as shown below.

A chiropractor from California who characterizes himself as a "holistic chiropractor" has written a book called *A Ten Minute Cure for the Common Cold*, which is packaged with an instructional video and sells for $59.95. An ad for the book calls his method a new-age scientific breakthrough based on 10 years of research into "nature's secrets." According to the ad, the secret for curing the common cold is mechanical finger pressure or light-thrust stimulation of the "bladder meridian energy point" that parallels the spinal column.

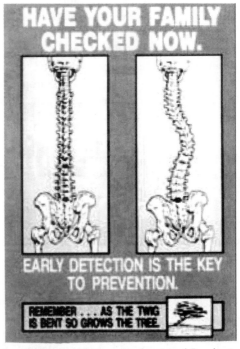

Poster from a recent Parker Professional Products catalog.

Such quasi-scientific terms might fool a medically ignorant public, but the claims should be regarded as flat-out quackery. No cure for the common cold is known to science. Some studies have found some benefit from an antiviral agent sprayed into the nose for certain cold viruses, and a few drugs have been found partially effective in treating influenza, another viral disease. The chiropractic profession has contributed nothing to the scientific management of respiratory infections.

Some chiropractic practice-builders advocate suggesting to patients that they are better but need lifetime periodic adjustments of their spine to maintain their health. Many patients can be persuaded to return for visits to chiropractors week after week because people who feel better tend to believe whatever explanation they receive from the person who treats them.

Chiropractors would like you to believe that what Smith described in his book is outdated and that very few chiropractors engage in the type of "brainwashing" he described. The Parker Seminars—which are still going strong and typically draw large audiences—provide detailed instructions for persuading patients to tell others to try chiropractic care for virtually every health problem they have. Parker Professional Products, which has been supplying chiropractors since 1951, offers a plethora of practice-building aids, including:

- "Chiropractic: A Step Toward Better Health" [welcome mat]
- "Childhood Fevers" [flier that "helps parents understand why their children have fevers, and the inadequacies of antibiotic therapy"]
- "Ear Infections" [flier to enable parents to "understand how subluxations can result in lowered resistance"]
- "Pregnancy" [flier about "the importance of chiropractic care throughout pregnancy, and for the newborn"]
- "Subluxations Are Often Present in Pain, Sickness, Death. Chiropractors Correct Subluxations" [poster]
- "How to Double Your Practice" [videotape]
- "Chiropractic is a way of life" [wall plaque]

- "Medicine treats the disease that has the person. Chiropractic treats the person who has the disease" [wall plaque]
- "Chiropractic relieves pain, restores health, prolongs life" [wall plaque]
- "The nervous system controls and coordinates ALL organs and structures of the human body" [wall plaque]
- "Make life a lot healthier for family and friends. Recommend chiropractic care" [wall plaque]
- "Subluxation: A Disease Occurring Worldwide in Epidemic Proportions" [poster]
- "Develop the once-a-month chiropractic habit" [wall plaque]

"Spinal Screening"

On October 5, 2001, I attended a regional fair in Berlin, Connecticut, which had an attendance of 90,000. Each year, there has been a chiropractic exhibit. At this year's exhibit, fairgoers waited in long lines to be tested with a Spinal Analysis Machine (S.A.M.), the twin-scale device pictured on page 157. The person to be tested stands with one foot on the platform of each scale. In most cases, the person's weight is unequally distributed so that one platform is higher than the other and the body tilts in the other direction. The chiropractor then indicates that one shoulder is higher than the other and levels the shoulders according to parallel lines on the device. This causes the spine to curve, and a red "X" is diagrammed at the midcurve, supposedly indicating the location of a "vertebral subluxation" that presses on a nerve and can cause various health problems.

The chiropractor's booth included posters about "pinched nerves" and "chiropractic health maintenance." Another poster asked whether the patient suffered from asthma, depression, poor circulation, shortness of breath, ear infections, growing pains, low immunity, "children's disorders," or about 20 other problems and suggested that chiropractic could help them all.

The exhibit also displayed literature claiming, "Chiropractic care provides better communication with nerve systems to every cell, tissue, and organ in the body" and that chiropractic provides "better sleep, clearer thinking, a healthier world filled with happier people." One brochure described how a group of chiropractors set up adjusting tables on the sidewalks of New York City to offer spinal adjustments to rescue workers on the day after the World Trade Center tragedy. Another brochure offered a "no-charge special offer 1st visit, with a $10 donation to the Kentuckiana Children's Center." The visit, said to have a normal value of $225, would include a consultation and health history with the chiropractor; orthopedic, neurologic, and chiropractic examinations; spinal x-rays, if needed; and a doctor's report of findings.

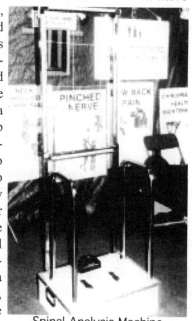

Spinal Analysis Machine at chiropractic exhibit.

S.A.M.'s manufacturer claims that 85% of people have "apparent differences" in leg length and suggests that use of the S.A.M. device can attract 20 to 40 new patients per week. The more likely explanation is that such "differences" are caused by slight variations of hip position or of normal spinal muscle tension. It is safe to assume that most of the people who are examined with the device are told they need further evaluation and that the "special-offer first visit" ends with a recommendation for months or even years of "treatment." All in all, the booth struck me as the modern equivalent of the 19th century snake-oil salesman.

Limits are Needed

Most people who consult chiropractors do so for low back pain. The fact that chiropractic thrusts produce "popping" sounds during spinal manipulation may impress patients that something highly therapeutic is taking place. Chiropractors have furthered their stature and patient confidence by having acquired the name of "doctor" and "physician," an accepted professional badge of integrity and trust. Although appropriate spinal manipulation may relieve symptoms in some cases, you should know that most cases of back pain resolve within a few weeks or months without treatment. You should also know that a substantial percentage of chiropractors will attempt to persuade everyone who consults them to return for periodic check-ups and "adjustments" throughout life. Yet no study has ever demonstrated that so-called "preventative maintenance" has any value for people who have no symptoms.

In recent years, with the rise of managed care, insurance companies are increasingly demanding that coverage be restricted to methods that have been proven cost-effective. If managed care companies require medical approval before chiropractic services are covered, chiropractic utilization will decrease sharply. Organized chiropractic has responded to this by insisting that chiropractors are qualified to practice independently and that they should be considered primary care providers. Many chiropractors state that they refer cases to medical doctors when needed and that they have sufficient diagnostic training to do so. However, because most common health problems lie outside of their scientifically supportable scope, seeing such patients would add unnecessary expense and delay appropriate care, even if proper referral takes place.

So far, at least, it seems that the chiropractic desire to be considered "primary care providers" has met with little success, but they are still generally permitted to see patients without medical referral.

17
The Chiropractic
Antitrust Suit

In 1976, Chester A. Wilk, DC, and several other chiropractors began a series of lawsuits against the American Medical Association (AMA), other professional organizations, and several individual critics, charging that they had conspired to destroy chiropractic and to illegally deprive chiropractors of access to laboratory, x-ray, and hospital facilities. Most of the defendant groups agreed in out-of-court settlements that their physician members were free to decide for themselves how to deal with chiropractors.

The main case against the AMA was first heard by a jury that decided in favor of the AMA, which, during the 1960s, had labeled chiropractic a "unscientific cult." A retrial, however, was allowed after an appeals court ruled that the original judge had improperly instructed the jury. A second trial was held before U.S. District Judge Susan Getzendanner. In 1987, Judge Getzendanner concluded that the AMA had engaged in an illegal boycott, and she issued an injunction forbidding certain things the organization had done. The judge's decision was appealed to the U.S. Supreme Court, which declined to hear the case and let it stand.

Many chiropractors trumpet the judge's ruling as an endorsement of what they do. However, it was not. The case was decided on narrow legal grounds (restraint of trade) and was not an evaluation of chiropractic methods. In fact, the full text of the judge's decision noted that during the 1960s, "there was a lot of material available to the AMA Committee on Quackery that supported its belief that all chiropractic was unscientific and deleterious." The judge also noted that chiropractors still took too many x-rays. She concluded that the dominant reason for the AMA's antichiropractic campaign was the belief that chiropractic was not in the best interest of patients. But she ruled that this did not justify attempting to contain and eliminate an entire licensed profession without first demonstrating that a less-restrictive campaign could not succeed in protecting the public.

To provide further information, here are two documents pertaining to this case. The first is the full text of the judge's permanent injunction order. (I have italicized sentences I believe are especially important.) The second is a brief comment on the case from the head of the AMA's law department.

Text of court order in *Wilk v. AMA*

In the United States District Court for the Northern District of Illinois Eastern Division
Chester A. Wilk, et al., plaintiffs, v. American Medical Association, et al., defendants
Permanent injunction order against AMA
Susan Getzendanner, District Judge

The court conducted a lengthy trial of this case in May and June of 1987 and on August 27, 1987, issued a 101 page opinion finding that the American Medical Association (AMA) and its members participated in a conspiracy against chiropractors in violation of the nation's antitrust laws. Thereafter, an opinion dated September 25, 1987, was substituted for the August 27, 1987, opinion. The question now before the court is the form of injunctive relief that the court will order.

As part of the injunctive relief to be ordered by the court against the AMA, the AMA shall be required to send a copy of this Permanent Injunction Order to each of its current members. The members of the AMA are bound by the terms of the Permanent Injunction Order if they act in concert with the AMA to violate the terms of the order. Accordingly, it is important that the AMA members understand the order and the reasons why the order has been entered.

The AMA's boycott and conspiracy

In the early 1960s, the AMA decided to contain and eliminate chiropractic as a profession. In 1963 the AMA's Committee on Quackery was formed. The committee worked aggressively — both overtly and covertly — to eliminate chiropractic. One of the principal means used by the AMA to achieve its goal was to make it unethical for medical physicians to professionally associate with chiropractors. Under Principle 3 of the AMA's Principles of Medical Ethics, it was unethical for a physician to associate with an "unscientific practitioner," and in 1966, the AMA's House of Delegates passed a resolution calling chiropractic an unscientific cult. To complete the circle, in 1967 the AMA's Judicial Council issued an opinion under Principle 3 holding that it was unethical for a physician to associate professionally with chiropractors.

The AMA's purpose was to prevent medical physicians from referring patients to chiropractors and accepting referrals of patients from chiropractors, to prevent chiropractors from obtaining access to hospital diagnostic services and membership on hospital medical staffs, to prevent medical physicians from teaching at chiropractic colleges or engaging in any joint research, and to prevent any cooperation between the two groups in the delivery of health care services.

The AMA believed that the boycott worked—that chiropractic would have achieved greater gains in the absence of the boycott. Since no medical physician would want to be considered unethical by his peers, the success of the boycott is not surprising. However, chiropractic achieved licensing in all 50 states during the existence of the Committee on Quackery.

The Committee on Quackery was disbanded in 1975 and some of the committee's activities became publicly known. Several lawsuits were filed by or on behalf of chiropractors and this case was filed in 1976.

Change in AMA position on chiropractic

In 1977, the AMA began to change its position on chiropractic. The AMA's Judicial Council adopted new opinions under which medical physicians could refer patients to chiropractors, but there was still the proviso that the medical physician should be confident that the services to be provided on referral would be performed in accordance with accepted scientific standards. In 1979, the AMA's House of Delegates adopted Report UU which said that not everything that a chiropractor may do is without therapeutic value, but it stopped short of saying that such things were based on scientific standards. It was not until 1980 that the AMA revised its Principles of Medical Ethics to eliminate Principle 3. Until Principle 3 was formally eliminated, there was considerable ambiguity about the AMA's position. The ethics code adopted in 1980 provided that a medical physician "shall be free to choose whom to serve, with whom to associate, and the environment in which to provide medical services."

The AMA settled three chiropractic lawsuits by stipulating and agreeing that under the current opinions of the Judicial Council a physician may, without fear of discipline or sanction by the AMA, refer a patient to a duly licensed chiropractor when he believes that referral may benefit the patient. The AMA confirmed that a physician may also choose to accept or to decline patients sent to him by a duly licensed chiropractor. Finally, the AMA confirmed that a physician may teach at a chiropractic college or seminar. These settlements were entered into in 1978, 1980, and 1986.

The AMA's present position on chiropractic, as stated to the court, is that it is ethical for a medical physician to professionally associate with chiropractors provided the physician believes that such association is in the best interests of his patient. This position has not previously been communicated by the AMA to its members.

Antitrust laws

Under the Sherman Act, every combination or conspiracy in restraint of trade is illegal. The court has held that the conduct of the AMA and its members constituted a conspiracy in restraint of trade based on the following facts: the purpose of the boycott was to eliminate chiropractic; chiropractors are in competition with some medical physicians; the boycott had substantial anti-competitive effects; there were no pro-competitive effects of the boycott; and the plaintiffs were injured as a result of the conduct. These facts add up to a violation of the Sherman Act.

In this case, however, the court allowed the defendants the opportunity to establish a "patient care defense" which has the following elements: (1) that they genuinely entertained a concern for what they perceive as scientific method in the care of each person with whom they have entered into a doctor-patient relationship; (2) that this concern is objectively reasonable; (3) that this concern has been the dominant motivating factor in the defendants' promulgation of Principle 3 and in the conduct intended to implement it; and (4) that this concern for scientific method in patient care could not have been adequately satisfied in a manner less restrictive of competition.

The court concluded that the AMA had a genuine concern for scientific methods in patient care, and that this concern was the dominant factor motivating the AMA's conduct. However, the AMA failed to establish that throughout the entire period of the boycott, from 1966 to 1980, this concern was objectively reasonable. The court reached that conclusion on the basis of extensive testimony from both witnesses for the plaintiffs and the AMA that some forms of chiropractic treatment are effective and the fact that the AMA recognized that chiropractic began to change in the early 1970s. Since the boycott was not formally over until Principle 3 was eliminated in 1980, the court found that the AMA was unable to establish that during the entire period of the conspiracy its position was objectively reasonable. Finally, the court ruled that the AMA's concern for scientific method in patient care could have been adequately satisfied in a manner less restrictive of competition and that a nationwide conspiracy to eliminate a *licensed* profession was not justified by the concern for scientific method. On the basis of these findings, the court concluded that the AMA had failed to establish the patient care defense.

None of the court's findings constituted a judicial endorsement of chiropractic. All of the parties to the case, including the plaintiffs and the AMA, agreed that chiropractic treatment of diseases such as diabetes, high blood pressure, cancer, heart disease and infectious disease is not proper, and that the historic theory of chiropractic, that there is a single cause and cure of disease, was wrong. There was disagreement between the parties as to whether chiropractors should engage in diagnosis. *There was evidence that the chiropractic theory of subluxations was unscientific, and evidence that some chiropractors engaged in unscientific practices.* The court did not reach the question of whether chiropractic theory was in fact scientific. However, the evidence in the case was that some forms of chiropractic manipulation of the spine and joints was therapeutic. AMA witnesses, including the present Chairman of the Board of Trustees of the AMA, testified that some forms of treatment by chiropractors, including manipulation, can be therapeutic in the treatment of conditions such as back pain syndrome.

Need for injunctive relief

Although the conspiracy ended in 1980, there are lingering effects of the illegal boycott and conspiracy which require an injunction. Some medical physicians' individual decisions on whether or not to professionally associate with a chiropractor are still affected by the boycott. The injury to chiropractors' reputations which resulted from the boycott has not been repaired. Chiropractors suffer current economic injury as a result of the boycott. The AMA has never affirmatively acknowledged that there are and should be no collective impediments to professional association and cooperation between chiropractors and medical physicians, except as provided by law. Instead, the AMA has consistently argued that its conduct has not violated the antitrust laws.

Most importantly, the court believes that it is important that the AMA members be made aware of the present AMA position that it is ethical for a medical physician to be professionally associated with a chiropractor if the physician believes it is in the best interest of his patient, so that the lingering effects of the illegal group boycott against chiropractors finally can be dissipated.

Under the law, every medical physician, institution, and hospital has the right to make an individual decision as to whether or not that physician, institution, or hospital shall associate professionally with chiropractors. Individual choice by a medical physician voluntarily to associate professionally with chiropractors should be governed only by restrictions under state law, if any, and by the individual medical physician's personal judgment as to what is in the best interest of a patient or patients. Professional association includes referrals, consultations, group practice in partnerships, Health Maintenance Organizations, Preferred Provider

Organizations, and other alternative health care delivery systems; the provision of treatment privileges and diagnostic services (including radiological and other laboratory facilities) in or through hospital facilities; association and cooperation in education programs for students in chiropractic colleges; and cooperation in research, health care seminars, and continuing education programs.

An injunction is necessary to assure that the AMA does not interfere with the right of a physician, hospital or other institution to make an individual decision on the question of professional association.

Form of injunction

1. The AMA, its officers, agents and employees, and all persons who act in active concert with any of them and who receive actual notice of this order are hereby permanently enjoined from restricting, regulating or impeding, or aiding and abetting others from restriction, regulating or impeding, the freedom of any AMA member or any institution or hospital to make an individual decision as to whether or not that AMA member, institution, or hospital shall professionally associate with chiropractors, chiropractic students, or chiropractic institutions.

2. *The Permanent Injunction does not and shall not be construed to restrict or otherwise interfere with the AMA's right to take positions on any issue, including chiropractic, and to express or publicize those positions, either alone or in conjunction with others.* Nor does this Permanent Injunction restrict or otherwise interfere with the AMA's right to petition or testify before any public body on any legislative or regulatory measure or to join or cooperate with any other entity in so petitioning or testifying. The AMA's membership in a recognized ac-

crediting association or society shall not constitute a violation of this Permanent Injunction.

3. The AMA is directed to send a copy of this order to each AMA member and employee, first class mail, postage prepaid, within thirty days of the entry of this order. In the alternative, the AMA shall provide the Clerk of the Court with mailing labels so that the court may send this order to AMA members and employees.

4. The AMA shall cause the publication of this order in *JAMA* and the indexing of the order under "Chiropractic" so that persons desiring to find the order in the future will be able to do so.

5. The AMA shall prepare a statement of the AMA's present position on chiropractic for inclusion in the current reports and opinions of the Judicial Council with an appropriate heading that refers to professional association between medical physicians and chiropractors, and indexed in the same manner that other reports and opinions are indexed. The court imposes no restrictions on the AMA's statement but only requires that it be consistent with the AMA's statement of its present position to the court.

6. The AMA shall file a report with the court evidencing compliance with this order on or before January 10, 1988.

It is so ordered.
Susan Getzendanner
United States District Judge
September 27, 1987

The AMA complied by publishing the judge's decision accompanied by the following statement by the AMA general counsel:

In the Wilk case, several chiropractors alleged that the AMA's former ethical guidelines violated the federal antitrust laws. The AMA defended the case on the ground that our positions on chiropractic were based on a genuine concern for patients—not on a desire for economic gain. District Judge Susan Getzendanner agreed. She found that the AMA had a genuine concern for scientific methods in patient care and that this concern was the dominant factor in motivating the AMA's conduct. Judge Getzendanner also found that the AMA's ethical guidelines have complied with the antitrust laws since 1980. Nevertheless, she concluded that an injunction was proper because old AMA statements on chiropractic might continue to have "lingering effects" injurious to chiropractors. Accordingly, she required the AMA to publish the order reproduced below. The Court of Appeals affirmed her decision.

The AMA's current position on chiropractic is clear. Paragraph 3.08 of the Current Opinions of the Council on Ethical and Judicial Affairs states that, "It is ethical for a physician to associate professionally with chiropractors provided that the physician believes that such association is in the best interests of his or her patient." In other words, each physician is free to make an individual decision whether and under what conditions to make or accept referrals, to teach in chiropractic schools, or otherwise to associate with chiropractors.

By the same token, neither professional ethics, the law, nor the court's injunction *requires* any physician to associate with or make referrals to chiropractors. Indeed, Judge Getzendanner declined, in her words, "to force a marriage" between medicine and chiropractic. Moreover, she refused to order changes in the Joint Commission's standards concerning the governance of hospital medical staffs. She concluded that "patient care in acute care hospitals ought to be under the control of fully licensed physicians rather than limited licensed practitioners." Finally, nothing in the court's injunction restrains the AMA or any state or local medical society from speaking out on any health care practice or issue, including chiropractic.

As noted above, this publication of the court's 1987 order ends the *Wilk* litigation. The AMA is pleased that this litigation has finally been concluded.

Although chiropractors hailed the antitrust suit verdict as an endorsement of chiropractic, it was not. The judge's verdict merely banned medical organizations from ordering their members not to professionally associate with chiropractors. (Individual doctors could still decide for themselves whether such association would serve the interests of their patients.)

On the other hand, the court made some rather damaging findings regarding chiropractic in the statement that "all of the parties to the case . . . agreed that chiropractic treatment of diseases such as diabetes, high blood pressure, cancer, heart disease and infectious disease is not proper, and that the historic theory of chiropractic, that there is a single cause and cure of a disease is wrong." The report mentioned, as noted previously, "there was evidence that the chiropractic theory of subluxation was unscientific, and evidence that some chiropractors engage in unscientific practices." Further, Judge Getzendanner concluded that "patient care in acute care hospitals ought to be under the care of fully licensed physicians rather than limited licensed practitioners." Finally, the court concluded that the AMA had a genuine concern for scientific methods in patient care and that this concern was a dominant factor motivating the AMA's conduct. In this regard, the AMA or any state or local medical society was free to speak out on any health care practice or issue, including chiropractic.

It is unfortunate that the *Wilk v. AMA* decision was based only on antitrust considerations. It would have been much more meaningful if the deciding factor had been whether the AMA had been correct in labeling subluxation-based chiropractic as an unscientific cult.

18
The AHCPR
Guideline

In December 1994, the Agency for Health Care Policy and Research (AHCPR), an agency of the U.S. Department of Health and Human Services, issued a booklet of guidelines for detecting and managing various types of acute low back pain in people age 18 and older [1]. The panel defined back problems as "activity intolerance due to back-related symptoms" and acute as "limitations of less than three months duration." The recommended guidelines were based mostly on a review of the scientific literature.

The 23-member expert panel included 11 medical doctors, two chiropractors (including Scott Haldeman, DC, MD, PhD), two osteopathic physicians, a psychologist, a nurse, a physical therapist, a minister, and others.

The guidelines focused on how to help patients improve their activity tolerance when impaired by uncomplicated back pain or back-related leg pain (sciatica). By uncomplicated condition, the panel meant that there was no serious underlying problem, such as a spinal tumor, infection, fracture, or indication that a nerve was in danger of being crushed by nearby structures. The panel concluded:

> Once the clinician has ruled out red flags and nonspinal pathology, the symptoms can be categorized as either sciatica or nonspecific back pain. In the absence of red flags, neither routine nor special testing is required in the first month of symptoms for either category. Most of these patients will recover spontaneously from their limitation of activities within one month.

The treatments that were analyzed included bed rest, various painkillers, nonsteroidal anti-inflammatory agents (NSAIDS), heat, cold, exercise, transcutaneous electrical nerve stimulation (TENS), shoe lifts, corsets, diathermy, belts, traction, steroidal facet injections, acupuncture, and spinal manipulation. Page iii of the panel's 172-page report summarized its findings:

Findings and recommendations on the assessment and treatment of adults with acute low back pain problems — activity limitations due to symptoms in the low back and/or back-related leg symptoms of less than 3 months' duration — are presented in this clinical practice guideline. The following are the principal conclusions of this guideline:

- The initial assessment of patients with acute low back problems focuses on the detection of "red flags" (indicators of potentially serious spinal pathology or other nonspinal pathology).
- In the absence of red flags, imaging studies and further testing of patients are not usually helpful during the first 4 weeks of low back symptoms.
- Relief of discomfort can be accomplished most safely with nonprescription medication and/or spinal manipulation.
- While some activity modification may be necessary during the acute phase, bed rest for more than 4 days is not helpful and may further debilitate the patient.
- Low-stress aerobic activities can be safely started in the first 2 weeks of symptoms to help avoid debilitation; exercises to condition trunk muscles are commonly delayed at least 2 weeks.
- Patients recovering from acute low back problems are encouraged to return to work or their normal daily activities as soon as possible.
- If low back symptoms persist, further evaluation may be indicated.

- Patients with sciatica may recover more slowly, but further evaluation can also be safely delayed.
- Within the first 3 months of low back symptoms, only patients with evidence of serious spinal pathology or severe, debilitating symptoms of sciatica, and physiologic evidence of specific nerve root compromise corroborated on imaging studies can be expected to benefit from surgery.
- With or without surgery, 80 percent of patients with sciatica recover eventually.
- Nonphysical factors (such as psychological or socioeconomic problems) may be addressed in the context of discussing reasonable expectations for recovery.

The major interest to chiropractors was the statement about spinal manipulation, which they hailed as an endorsement of chiropractic. However, it was not. It merely supports the use of manipulation in carefully selected patients. Only a few of the research studies on which its conclusions were based involved manipulation by chiropractors; most were done by medical doctors and physical therapists whose practices are not identical to those of chiropractors. The word chiropractic does not even appear in the body of the report. Moreover, Dr. Stephen Barrett, who is the leading medical authority on the chiropractic marketplace, has noted that the research studies do not reflect what often happens in practice outside of research settings:

Most chiropractors manipulate the vast majority of patients who walk through their door, some use techniques that have not been studied scientifically, and many urge all of their patients to undergo monthly or even weekly "preventive maintenance" visits throughout their life. In addition, many chiropractors emphasize a technique that is more vigorous (and therefore less safe) than the controlled manipulation used by other practitioners [2].

The panel's evaluation of the effectiveness of manipulation was based primarily on a meta-analysis that was summarized in the October 1992 issue of the *Annals of Internal Medicine* [3]. This study, conducted by the Rand Corporation, was funded by a $1 million grant from the California Chiropractic Foundation. Some 112 articles were reviewed by the agency. Only 13 were found acceptable; among them, 9 were reported by Paul Shekelle, MD, who headed the project. The two studies that he believed were most significant found, strangely, that spinal manipulation was effective only between the 14th and 28th days from the onset of pain. The explanation for this finding raises serious questions and casts doubt on the statistical validity of the studies.

A subsequent study conducted in Helsinki, Finland, and reported in the *New England Journal of Medicine* [4] casts doubt on the value of stretching the back structures during this healing period. The Helsinki report subjected patients with low back pain to a program of bending to either side, and backwards and forwards to tolerance of pain, 10 times every hour during the day and then comparing the recovery times with those of a control group encouraged to go about their usual activities of daily living to tolerance. The patients who engaged in back stretching and twisting took longer to recover than the controls did, which suggests that undue back motion, including spinal manipulation, can delay recovery. From these additional studies, the best treatment for ordinary acute low back pain can be summarized as, "Leave the back alone and in 4 weeks it will be healed. If healing does not occur, search for other trouble—a red flag like a ruptured disk or spinal tumor."

References

1. Bigos S and others. Clinical Practice Guideline #14, Acute Low Back Problems in Adults. Rockville MD: Agency for Health Care Policy and Research, December 1994.
2. Barrett S. Don't let chiropractors fool you. Quackwatch Web site, 2000.
3. Shekelle PG. Spinal manipulation for low back pain. Annals of Internal Medicine, October 1992.
4. Malmivaara A and others. The treatment of acute low back pain: Bed rest, exercises, or ordinary activity? New England Journal of Medicine 332:351–355, 1995.

19
Some Notes on a Leading
Chiropractic Textbook

Following my visit to New York Chiropractic College, Louis Sportelli, DC, a leading spokesperson for his profession, sent me literature and the second edition of *Principles and Practice of Chiropractic,* which is considered one of chiropractic's most comprehensive and authoritative textbooks. Published in 1992 by Appleton & Lange, the book was edited by Scott Haldeman, DC, MD, PhD, a third-generation chiropractor who is associate clinical professor of neurology at the University of California-Irvine and also an adjunct professor at Los Angeles Chiropractic College.

The book has four sections: "History, Philosophy and Sociology of Chiropractic," "Physiological and Biomechanical Principles," "Spinal Analysis and Diagnostic Methods," and "Chiropractic Care."

The section on history, philosophy, and sociology of chiropractic constitutes about 10% of the book's pages and 20% of its chapters. Noting that it is unusual for a professional textbook to devote so much space to such topics, Haldeman adds that "these topics are likely to remain an intricate part of every chiropractic student's education." The section traces chiropractic's origin to the case of Harvey Lillard, a supposedly deaf janitor who on September 8, 1895, was allegedly cured of his deafness when Daniel David Palmer, an Iowa grocer-turned-magnetic-healer, administered the first chiropractic thrust on Lillard's back and became the "Father of Chiropractic." The book relates the trials and tribulations of chiropractors and their theory, including Palmer's jailing for 15 days for practicing medicine without a license. After describing key developments up to the time the book was published, one chapter author (a former chiropractic college president) concludes: "The extent to which chiropractic has been, or is, a cult would be an interesting research topic."

The second section addresses the basis of chiropractic itself in a potpourri of correctly described anatomical features of the spine, but without demonstrating a rational model of subluxation theory. It describes the effects of nerve compression but does not specify what compresses the nerve or how this could be related to disease. No description of an anatomical "subluxation" amenable to manipulation occurs in the entire book. Yet a chapter is written on how spinal lesions could theoretically affect visceral organs by "smooth visceral reflex" and how these diseased organs can be relieved by manipulations. The chapter also mentions experiments in which beta-endorphins, the body's own opiate-like hormones, increase after manipulation. Even if this is true, endorphins should then also be increased from manipulation of a foot or any part of the body. At most, endorphins may temporarily relieve pain. Like morphine, they heal nothing.

The third section describes spinal analysis and diagnostic methods. A few pages cover history-taking and physical examination as done by medical doctors. However, since most chiropractors know little about disease, how to recognize it, and how to treat it, these diagnostic procedures would seem to have little or no practical purpose. Many pages are devoted to methods of physical examination and instrument-testing that are not taught in medical schools.

One piece of laboratory apparatus described in the book is a spirometer. Its use is correctly described as a simple test that quickly measures the breathing capacity of patients with asthma and other respiratory diseases. However, there is no scientific evidence that spinal manipulation is effective against asthma. Medical science, on the other hand, has made great strides in discovering factors that trigger asthmatic attacks, such as allergies to dust mites and various foods. As the factors involved in asthmatic attacks have become clear, effective drugs have been developed based on an understanding of the mechanisms involved. In contrast to hypothetical chiropractic procedures, medical science has revealed the true nature of asthma and has produced effective treatments. In comparison, chiropractic has discovered nothing and knows little of the basics—yet uses spirometry and spinal manipulations nevertheless.

During the past 100 years, medical doctors have made tremendous strides in the diagnosis of thousands of diseases and their causes, as evidenced in standard medical texts and journals. The paucity of information in Haldeman's book provides no reason to rely on chiropractors for diagnosis.

The fourth section of the textbook deals with chiropractic care. My overall impression from reading what it says about chiropractic's manipulative maneuvers is that their effects are entirely hypothetical. Chiropractors don't seem to know what is being manipulated and what occurs as a result. In other words, they do not know exactly what they are doing. Haldeman basically admits this on page 454, where he asks, "What is one trying to achieve by spinal adjustment?" His candid answer is: "Unfortunately, far more is speculated than is truly and scientifically known about the mechanism of action of a manipulation or an adjustment."

Another example of the difference between medical science and chiropractic is the amount of discussion devoted to the speculative cause and treatment of headache. The book contains only one short paragraph on this subject, in which a number of treatment outcome studies "showing some value" are listed. In contrast, a leading medical textbook, the 20th edition of *Cecil's Textbook of Medicine*, devotes six detailed pages to headache and describes the cause, pathology, prognosis, and treatment of some 30 types of headaches such as migraine, brain tumors, subdural hematoma, glaucoma, and sinusitis, none of which are described in any detail by Haldeman.

The Cecil text also mentions a tension type headache that may grip the whole head like a vise. It is this type of headache that chiropractic claims to relieve by "adjusting subluxations" in the neck. Many of these patients, states Cecil, are anxious and depressed and may respond to appropriate antidepressant medication— which, of course, chiropractors are not qualified or licensed to prescribe.

Haldeman's text can also be compared with the recently published *Essentials of Musculoskeletal Care*, a 755-page work distributed by the American Medical Association. This book does not mention "vertebral subluxations" or recommend spinal manipulation as a treatment.

A chapter in Haldeman's text by John J. Triano, DC, describes the chiropractic "subluxation" as a hypothetical concept with multiple definitions, thereby admitting that no clear-cut anatomical abnormality exists. However, Triano substitutes the term "functional spinal lesion (FSL)," the definition of which appears to be just as nebulous.

In another chapter, a dean and a professor at Palmer College say this about chiropractic's future:

> If continued scientific investigation of chiropractic were to elucidate the underlying principles, would such an undertaking undermine chiropractic's philosophical tenants and destroy the identity of the discipline and so the discipline itself? Must chiropractic be prepared to abandon its philosophy and identity, to adapt to scientific discoveries? These questions, of course, cannot be answered with certainty.

Judged by scientific medical standards, this has already happened. Chiropractic, as defined in terms of "subluxation," does not exist. The public interest would be served if chiropractors admitted that their theory is false, abandoned it, and devoted their energy to figuring out what they do that may be useful.

20
Complaints against Chiropractors

Chiropractors have long claimed that there are more complaints against medical doctors than there are against chiropractors. They have used anecdotal evidence and testimonials almost exclusively to promote their cause. They point with pride to patient satisfaction, while, at the same time, criticize medical doctors for using "dangerous" drugs and surgery.

Their claims for fewer complaints against chiropractors may not be true, at least on a percentage basis in Connecticut, where in 1997 I found that there were 276 complaints against 9,707 medical doctors versus 23 complaints against 648 licensed chiropractors. Percentagewise, this means there were more complaints against chiropractors, 3.55%, versus 2.88% against medical doctors. The following example of a patient complaint appears in the records of the Connecticut State Board of Chiropractic Examiners.

The patient was treated for chronic migraine headaches by a chiropractor who advised that he could cure her headaches and acne. During her first visit, she underwent standing and sitting full-spine x-ray examinations, which, she was advised, were done to enable her treatment progress to be monitored.

One part of her "treatment" was a "coccygeal-meningeal procedure," during which the chiropractor inserted his hand into her rectum to examine and manipulate it. This procedure was administered on at least five occasions.

Upon learning that the patient was planning to take a trip in a pressurized airliner, the chiropractor advised her to self-administer this procedure while in flight. She was instructed that the pressurized cabin would allow her to safely perform the procedure herself. The chiropractor gave her a rubber glove for this purpose and stated that the procedure was necessary for proper chiropractic "adjustment."

When the patient refused to continue with the procedure, the chiropractor said that he could not continue to treat her. Nevertheless, he did so for several months.

The patient's husband was also treated. He, too, underwent full-spinal x-ray examinations and was advised to have the rectal procedure. He refused the treatment, however, and terminated his relationship. The chiropractor asked him to sign a form relieving the chiropractor of all responsibility and liability, but the husband refused to sign and filed a complaint with the chiropractic licensing board. The board concluded:

- No known manipulative technique is effective for treating acne, and that the chiropractor's statement in this regard constitutes material deception, as alleged.
- The chiropractor excessively x-rayed the patient by taking full-spine films on three different occasions; this constituted incompetent practice.
- Rectal manipulation was not taught in any college of chiropractic approved by the board, and constituted illegal conduct.

The board, in effect, ruled that there should be scientific proof of a chiropractic procedure and, in referring to the rectal manipulation, stated "this approach is considered experimental and lacking current substantiation in the scientific literature." It is of interest that the board made such a finding when the whole chriopractic "subluxation" theory lacks scientific proof.

The board found the chiropractor guilty of a number of charges and made the following disposition:

The chiropractor's license to practice chiropractic is suspended for a period of one year and he is ordered to pay a civil penalty of $5,000. The period of suspension shall commence 45 days from the date of the mailing of this decision. The civil penalty shall be payable to the State of Connecticut. The respondent is also placed on a probationary status for a period of three years. During the period of probation, he must report on each patient he has x-rayed, the dates of the x-rays and the precise views taken.

Similar stories of weird treatments undoubtedly can be found among the medical profession as well, but there is good reason to believe that they are far more common among chiropractors. A few hundred medical doctors have embraced the homeopathic notion that "remedies" so dilute that they contain no molecules of the original "active" substance can exert powerful therapeutic effects. Other doctors use chelation therapy and all sorts of other dubious "alternative" medical treatments. However, legitimate health professions do not have a senseless underlying theory but are based on the commonly shared knowledge of health and disease. Thus, unscientific practices are not widely taught in medical schools, as they are in chiropractic schools. Moreover, chiropractic schools attract students who are more prone to misbeliefs. Many have been "raised in chiropractic" and come to school with deep-seated beliefs that health and illness are centered around the spine.

For these reasons—and more—I believe that complaints and malpractice suits against chiropractors will grow exponentially as the silliness of subluxation theory becomes more widely realized.

Insurance Fraud and Abuse

Chiropractors also appear to be involved in an undue number of cases of insurance fraud and abuse. A prominent example is the case of chiropractors Steven Verchow and Alexander Kuntzevich, who, doing business as V&K, operated a string of clinics in New Jersey. In 1987, according to one press report, they began treating people for "auto accident injuries that were never inflicted, and pain and suffering never endured." Between 1987 and 1992, they collected $12 million from a state insurance fund and had billed out for $40 million more.

According to press reports, chiropractors at their Accident and Illness Center in Passaic saw an average of 100 patients in an 8-hour shift. One doctor, who was dubbed "The Fastest Examiner in the West," allegedly did complex orthopedic evaluations on 222 patients in a single day and billed $45,256 for that work. His examinations, some of his colleagues said, lasted mere seconds. Another of the chiropractors was called "Dirty Harry." He moved about the corridors in a blood-stained lab coat. His patients could be heard screaming from behind closed examining room doors. He reportedly billed as much as $100,000 in a day. Many of the patients were generated by arranging for carloads of poor immigrants to crash into each other at speeds not exceeding 4 miles per hour. The cars were barely damaged, but all passengers allegedly acquired whiplash injuries, with pain and suffering to follow.

These descriptions come from depositions by doctors and patients during New Jersey's investigation of what law enforcement authorities described as the biggest auto insurance scam in state history up to that time. For this, the chiropractors were fined $750,000, surrendered their claim to the $40 million, and were suspended from practice for at least 5 years.

Although some "personal injury mills" involve medical doctors as well, chiropractors appear to be proportionally more involved and often instigate the MD/DC schemes.

21
Recent Studies on Tension Headaches, Low Back Pain, Asthma, and Colic

Since publication of the first edition of this book, four important controlled studies of chiropractic therapy have been published in major medical journals.

The first of these compared the effect of active and simulated spinal manipulation on 80 children receiving medical treatment for asthma [1]. In this study, medical care with inhalant drugs was continued along with the "adjustments," because it was considered unethical to discontinue the drug therapy. The findings and conclusion were clear and unequivocal: "In children with mild or moderate asthma, the addition of chiropractic manipulation to usual medical care provided no benefit." The study should put to rest the false chiropractic claims that spinal manipulation is an effective treatment for asthma.

The second study compared the effect on low back pain of spinal manipulation, a physical therapy (using an exercise program called the McKenzie method), and no therapy (merely giving patients an educational booklet) [2]. The study involved 321 adults. The cost per person was $429 for chiropractic, $437 for physical therapy, and $153 for the booklet. The researchers concluded:

> For patients with low back pain, the McKenzie method of physical therapy and chiropractic manipulation had similar effects and costs, and the patients had only marginal better outcomes than those receiving the minimal intervention of an educational booklet. Whether the limited benefits of these treatments are worth the additional costs is open to question.

In an accompanying editorial, Paul Shekelle, MD, of the Rand Corporation, added, "There appears to be little evidence to support the use of spinal manipulation for non-musculoskeletal conditions." Referring the the fact that neck manipulation can cause a stroke, Shekelle also states that "the use of cervical manipulation arouses far greater concern about safety than the use of lumbar manipulation." [3]

The third study, which involved 75 adults, compared the effect of chiropractic neck manipulation, bed rest, exercise, and ordinary activity on tension headaches. The researchers concluded that return to ordinary activity was superior to either of the other treatments and that "as an isolated intervention, spinal manipulation does not seem to have a positive effect on episodic tension-type headache." [4]

The fourth study examined the effect of chiropractic manipulation on infants with colic and found no benefit [5].

Three of the aforementioned studies tested claims based on chiropractic "subluxation" theory, and their results support the core challenge and conclusion of this book: that *subluxation-based chiropractic is a hoax.* The back-pain study data even challenge whether manipulation is effective or cost-effective for treating back pain.

References

1. Balon J and others: A comparison of active and simulated chiropractic manipulation as adjunctive treatment for childhood asthma. New England Journal of Medicine 339:1013–1020, 1998.
2. Cherkin DC and others. A comparison of physical therapy, chiropractic manipulation, and provision of an educational booklet for the treatment of patients with low back pain. New England Journal of Medicine 339:1021–1029, 1998.
3. Shekelle PG. What role for chiropractic in health care? New England Journal of Medicine 339:1074–1075, 1998.
4. Bove G, Nilsson N. Spinal manipulation in the treatment of episodic tension-type headache: A randomized controlled trial. JAMA 280:1576–1579, 1998.
5. Olafsdottir E and others. Randomised controlled trial of infantile colic treated with chiropractic spinal manipulation. Archives of Diseases in Childhood 84:138–141, 2001.

22
Final Comments

This book's conclusion—that chiropractic, as defined, is a hoax—has been expressed by others many times before. Yet, despite this, chiropractic has flourished to the extent that as many as 70,000 chiropractors in the United States are legally permitted practice this hoax in every state of the union.

Many chiropractors offer "nutritional counseling" and (improperly) prescribe dietary supplements and herbs in an apparent attempt to compensate for their inability to prescribe standard medications. A few, on the other hand, have renounced chiropractic's subluxation theory and limit their treatment to relieving stiff muscles and joints. This book's main thrust and purpose is to distinguish between scientific medical care based on proven facts and chiropractic care based on a metaphysical belief. Chiropractic has many devoted, hard-core believers, whereas medical care has the scientific proof of the greatest advances in health care in the history of humankind. This book highlights the difference between the two.

My friends, including physician colleagues and even chiropractors, have asked me, "Why are you so upset with chiropractic?" They reason that if people want to risk their life going to a quack, why not let them. It is, after all, a free country and if they want that type of care, they are free to make that choice.

It is admittedly difficult to deny freedom of choice as an inalienable right, especially in matters so vital as health, life, and death. However, chiropractic licensing carries with it the connotation of the approval by our government agencies. We have, for better or worse, many government regulations to pro-

185

tect consumers. I believe that if legislators license a hoax, consumers have a right to know that and to be informed by those who discern the truth.

It should be clear from reading this book that chiropractic is not based on science. Chiropractic "subluxations" do not press on nerves that interfere with energy going down those nerves, causing disease in the body's internal organs. It is, of course, almost impossible to prove this negatively to everyone's satisfaction. After all, thousands even believe in UFOs and, in regard to health, believe in all sorts of alternative, unproven health care claims.

The facts presented in this book should lead you to conclude that chiropractic's subluxation theory is a hoax, that back pain is not caused by "vertebral subluxations," and that any positive benefits from manipulation are not the result of "correcting subluxations."

Ian D. Coulter, PhD, a former president of Canadian Memorial Chiropractic College, has hinted at the inevitability of science debunking chiropractic. In the textbook *Principles and Practice of Chiropractic*, he stated, "The extent to which chiropractic has been, or is, a cult would be an interesting research topic." In another chapter of the textbook, a leading chiropractic historian wrote:

> If continued scientific investigation of chiropractic were to elucidate the underlying principles, would such an undertaking undermine chiropractic's philosophical tenants and destroy the identity of the discipline and the discipline itself? Must chiropractic be prepared to abandon its philosophy and its identity, to adapt to scientific discoveries?

Consumer Reports answered this question in 1975, loudly and clearly:

> Not a single scientific study in the 80 years existence of chiropractic or the entire history of medicine shows that manipulation can affect any of the basic life patterns.

But a vast amount of evidence suggests it cannot.

In 1895, neither D.D. Palmer (chiropractic's founder) nor his contemporaries could foresee that research. In the year 2001, however, there is no excuse for ignoring it. Unless most research in the 20th century is wrong, Palmer's disease theory belongs in the pages of 19th century history, along with bleeding, purging, and the other blind alleys of medicine.

I believe that chiropractors should admit that subluxation theory is a hoax and attempt to upgrade their colleges into scientific institutions patterned after medical schools, as the osteopaths have done. Until that happens, those who find chiropractic to be unscientific and unconscionable will surely continue to speak out—as is done in this book.

Is There a Solution?

Can chiropractic survive if it remains based on a false theory? And even if it can, would this serve the best interests of patients whose care is based on this theory? Might chiropractic be split into two parts, one that limits its care to evidence-based treatment of musculoskeletal problems and the other still ingrained "subluxation" concepts?

I believe that the best solution would be to mirror the practice of dentists, optometrists, and podiatrists, whose scope is sharply defined, but who practice independently. To do this, chiropractors would have to abandon subluxation theory and stop pretending that their scope is virtually unlimited. They would also have to restructure their educational programs so that they produce graduates who can clearly distinguish who is within their scope of practice and who is not.

During my visit to New York Chiropractic College, I suggested to the dean and to President Padgett that they (a) convert their handsome college into an accredited medical school and (b) abandon the false beliefs that spinal "adjustments" can treat disease and maintain wellness. I also sought the opinion of chiropractor Lester Lamm, dean of continuing education at Western States Chiropractic College in Portland, Oregon. Both deans firmly rejected such a suggestion, but dean Lamm sent information about the college that may indicate a trend toward conversion.

The college had instituted an "integrated" program intended to prepare chiropractors to be primary care physicians. The program was centered around two newly employed osteopathic physicians who would supervise a clinic where chiropractic students could learn aspects of standard medicine. The program, as described in the brochures, hardly constituted adequate training for managing the full range of patients who would be seen in a typical medical office—and I said this to the dean. He replied that it was as good as the training of nurses, physician's assistants, and nurse practitioners who function as primary care providers. Furthermore, he was not about to abandon chiropractic, which he insisted was a scientific practice.

Despite the denial of these two deans, any bridging of chiropractic and medicine will inevitably be based on a medical model of health and disease. Whether this can be done by (a) upgrading the current system, (b) affiliating with science-based universities or medical centers, or (c) converting chiropractic colleges into accredited medical schools, remains to be seen. But one thing is certain: As time goes on, the health marketplace will demand greater accountability. For chiropractic to survive, its practitioners will have to limit their scope to scientifically oriented physical therapy of musculoskeletal problems, improve the quality of their training, develop evidence-base treatment standards, and relegate the subluxation theory and its associated practices to the dust bin of history.

Part V

Appendices

Glossary
Where to Get Additional Information

Appendix A
Glossary

ACA. Abbreviation for American Chiropractic Association, the largest chiropractic professional organization.

Acute back pain. Back pain that lasts a short while, usually a few days to several weeks. Episodes lasting longer than 3 months are not considered acute.

Acute condition. Condition that has rapid onset and follows a short but relatively severe course.

"Adjustment." Term that most chiropractors use to describe whatever method(s) they use to correct spinal problems, whether by hand or with an instrument.

AHCPR back pain guideline. Report on the care of acute low back pain issued in 1994 by the Agency for Health Care Policy and Research.

"Alternative" health method. An unproven method that lacks a scientifically plausible rationale.

Applied kinesiology (AK). Pseudoscientific system of muscle-testing and therapy based on assertions that specific muscle weaknesses are signs of disease in body organs.

"Big Idea." The chiropractic concept that the body heals itself when interference to the proper functioning of the nervous system is removed.

Cauda equina. The bundle within the spinal canal comprised of all of spinal nerve roots below the first (top-most) lumbar vertebra.

Cervical. Pertaining to the neck, e.g., cervical vertebrae.

Chronic back pain. Back pain that lasts more than 3 months or recurs frequently.

192 Part V: Appendices

Clinical activities or subjects. Activities or subjects that involve patient care.

Contraindication. Reason that a diagnostic or therapeutic measure should not be used.

Controlled clinical trial. Research method in which people are assigned, under predetermined rules, to either an experimental group (which receives the treatment being tested) or a control group (which receives another treatment or a placebo). If subjects are randomly assigned, the result is a randomized clinical trial (RCT).

Cult. An unscientific system that involves devotion to a person, ideal, or philosophy. This description fits chiropractic's early years and is still applicable to subluxation-based chiropractic today.

DC. Abbreviation for "doctor of chiropractic."

Double-blind study. An experiment in which neither the experimental subjects nor those responsible for the treatment or data collection know which subjects receive the treatment being tested and which subjects receive something else (such as a placebo).

Foundation for Chiropractic Education and Research (FCER). ACA-affiliated organization that funds chiropractic research and distributes materials promoting chiropractic. Its publications include books and fliers that criticize antibiotic usage and recommend chiropractic treatment for childhood ear infections.

Herniated disk ("ruptured disk"). Protrusion of the central gelatinous material of an intervertebral disk through its outer fibrous cover.

Homeopathy. A pseudoscience based on the notion that diseases can be healed by administering tiny amounts of substances that, in large amounts, would cause healthy people to develop symptoms like those of the ailment treated.

Iatrogenic disease (or symptom). Any complication induced in a patient by a physician's actions or therapy.

ICA. Abbreviation for International Chiropractors Association, the second largest chiropractic professional organization.

Informed consent. Permission given by a patient who has been fully apprised of the nature and risks of a proposed treatment.

Innate Intelligence. An alleged inborn ability of the body to heal itself, which chiropractors believe is enhanced by spinal "adjustments."

Insurance abuse. Charging for services that are not medically necessary, do not conform to professionally recognized standards, or are unfairly priced.

Insurance fraud. Intentional deception or misrepresentation intended to result in an unauthorized insurance benefit.

Intervertebral disk. The tough cartilage that serves as a cushion between two vertebrae. Each disk has a gelatinous-like center that may protrude to form a disk herniation.

Lesion. Abnormal change in the structure of an organ or body tissue resulting from injury or disease, especially a change that is circumscribed and well defined. Examples are cuts, burns, skin eruptions, and tumors.

Lumbar vertebrae. The five bones in the lower-back portion of the spine.

Maintenance care. Subluxation-based program of periodic spinal examinations and "adjustments" alleged to help maintain the patient's health. Also called "preventive maintenance" or "preventative maintenance."

Manipulation. A forceful, high-velocity thrust that stretches a joint beyond its passive range of movement to increase its mobility. Manipulation is usually accompanied by an audible pop or click. Because of the speed involved, the patient does not have control and the potential for injury is greater than exists with mobilization.

Meric system. Chiropractic system based on the theory that specific spinal joints are associated with specific organs, requiring "adjustment" of certain vertebrae for certain diseases.

Mixer. Chiropractor who uses other modalities besides manual manipulation of the spine.

Mobilization. Method of manipulation, movement, or stretching to increase range of motion in muscles and joints that does not involve a high-velocity thrust.

Musculoskeletal. Relating to or involving bones, muscles, and/ or their attachments to other body structures.

National Association for Chiropractic Medicine (NACM). Reformist organization whose members have renounced chiropractic dogma and denounced the unscientific methods used by many of their colleagues.

Osteopathic physician. Graduate of an osteopathic medical school. Osteopathy was originally based on false beliefs similar to those of chiropractic but gradually abandoned them and incorporated the theories and practices of scientific medicine.

Practice-builders. Individuals or organizations that teach chiropractors how to increase their income through marketing techniques, increased productivity, creative billing, and/or other activities. The term has a negative connotation because many practice-building consultants have recommended methods that are unethical.

"Preventative maintenance." Term chiropractors use to describe periodic spinal examinations and correction of "subluxations." The usual frequency is monthly or weekly. There is no scientific evidence that this practice provides any health benefit.

Primary care provider. Health care professional who provides basic health services, manages routine health care needs, and is usually the first contact when someone needs care.

Pseudoscience. A theory or methodology that is represented as scientific but has no basis in reality. Its proponents typically use scientific terminology and concoct evidence (or distort scientific findings) in support of their beliefs.

Quackery. Promotion of an unproven health product or service, usually for personal gain.

"Raised in chiropractic." Having grown up in a family that deeply believes in subluxation theory and periodic spinal checkups and "adjustments."

Rand studies of manipulation. A series of reports published in the early 1990s about the appropriateness of spinal manipulation for low back pain. (The Rand Corporation, of Santa Monica, California, is a prominent nonprofit organization that does research in many fields.)

"Red flag." Warning sign that a procedure might be dangerous.

Reformist chiropractors. Chiropractors who limit their practice to conservative treatment for musculoskeletal conditions and have openly renounced chiropractic's subluxation theory and the unscientific procedures used by chiropractors.

Sacral. Pertaining to the sacrum (the triangular bone at the bottom of the spinal column).

Sciatic pain (sciatica). Pain in the lower back and hip radiating down the back of the thigh into the leg, usually caused by a herniated intervertebral disk.

Scoliosis. Abnormal lateral (sideward) curvature of the spine. Spinal manipulation may relieve discomfort associated with spinal stiffness but cannot influence the course of a scoliotic curve.

Self-limiting illness. Ailment that usually subsides without treatment.

SMT. Abbreviation for spinal manipulative therapy.

Spinal manipulation. See Manipulation.

Spinograph. A 14- by 36-inch x-ray film of the entire spine, usually taken with the patient standing, that chiropractors use to look for "subluxations."

Straight chiropractor. Chiropractor who clings to chiropractic's original doctrine that most health problems are caused by misaligned spinal bones ("vertebral subluxations") and are correctable by manual manipulation of the spine.

Subluxation. Medical term for partial dislocation of a bone. Chiropractors define "vertebral subluxation" in many ways.

Thoracic vertebrae. The 12 vertebrae in the thoracic or upper-back portion of the spine.

Vertebra. Bony segment of the spine that encircles and helps protect the spinal cord and nerves. The plural of vertebra is vertebrae.

Vertebral artery. Arteries, one on each side, that thread through holes in the six upper cervical vertebrae. Sudden rotation during neck manipulation can injure them and interrupt blood flow to the lower part of the brain, causing a stroke.

Vertebral subluxation complex. A "modern" chiropractic term for the chiropractic subluxation.

Viscera. The soft internal organs of the body, especially those contained within the abdomen and chest.

"Vital force." A term "alternative" practitioners use to describe a non-material force that enables the body to function and heal itself. (See Innate Intelligence.) The concept that living things function because of such a force is called *vitalism*.

"Yet disease." A technique for selling chiropractic care by asking people whether they have experienced various symptoms "yet."

Appendix B
Where to Get
Additional Information

Each of the following sources provides a significant amount of reliable information:

• *Bonesetting, Chiropractic, and Cultism* (1963), by Samuel Homola, DC: A thorough analysis of chiropractic's early history and the shortcomings of its theories and methods. Many of the problems still exist today.

• *Independent Practitioners under Medicare: A Report to Congress*, by Wilbur J. Cohen: An expert panel's assessment of the chiropractic marketplace during the 1960s.

• *At Your Own Risk: The Case against Chiropractic* (1969), by Ralph Lee Smith: A devastating exposé that describes the development of chiropractic and the shoddy salesmanship that characterized its practice during the 1960s.

• Chiropractors. *Consumer Reports* 59:383-390, 1994.

• *Chiropractic: The Victim's Perspective* (1995), by George Magner: A comprehensive report on chiropractic's history, current status, marketing tactics, dubious diagnostics and therapeutics, insurance abuses, dangers, and "chiropractic pediatrics."

• *Inside Chiropractic: A Patient's Guide* (1999), by Samuel Homola, DC: An incisive guide to chiropractic's history, benefits, and shortcomings. No one should ever contemplate or undergo chiropractic care without reading this book.

• Chirobase (http:www.chirobase.org), operated by Stephen Barrett, MD: Offers comprehensive information on chiropractic's history, theories, and current practices. Its contents include the full text of *Bonesetting, At Your Own Risk,* and

Independent Practitioners under Medicare. It provides detailed advice on how to choose a chiropractor and maintains a referral directory of chiropractors who seem trustworthy.

• *Essentials of Musculoskeletal Care*, 2nd edition, edited by Walter Greene, MD: A comprehensive medical textbook produced by the American Academy of Orthopaedic Surgeons and the American Academy of Pediatrics.

Index

New England Books
L.A. Chotkowski, M.D. F.A.C.P.
1143 Chamberlain Highway
Kensington, CT 06037
Tel. 860.828.5016
Email: DrChot@aol.com

2-19-03

Dear Dr. Beauvais, MD,

Thanks for helping to
spread the word.
If you find the
book effective, perhaps
you might suggest your
library to carry it.
yours,

L. A. Chotkowski